BRAIN AND DISSOCIATED MIND

BRAIN AND DISSOCIATED MIND

PETR BOB

Nova Biomedical Books
New York

LIBRARY OF CONGRESS CATALOGING-IN-PUBLICATION DATA

Available upon request.

ISBN 978-1-60692-035-0

Published by Nova Science Publishers, Inc. ✛ New York

CONTENTS

Preface		**vii**
Chapter 1	Conscious and Subliminal Mind	**1**
Chapter 2	History of Dissociation and Its Present Times	**7**
Chapter 3	Dissociation and Schizophrenia	**33**
Chapter 4	Dissociation and "Wounded Mind"	**39**
Chapter 5	Pain, Dissociation and Subliminal Consciousness	**49**
Chapter 6	Dissociation and Dreaming Brain	**63**
Chapter 7	Brain and Consciousness	**73**
Chapter 8	Chaos, Self-Organization and Dissociated Mind	**79**
Chapter 9	Consciousness Experienced but Unexplained	**89**
References		**95**
Index		**135**

PREFACE

BOOK DESCRIPTION

This book presents current knowledge regarding relationship between conscious and unconscious processes in the human mind and dissociation between them, in a close relationship with modern neuroscientific research. Following the framework of traditional psychological and psychiatric terms proposed by Janet and developed also by Freud and Jung, the author shows new connections between modern theoretical neuroscience and psychological concept of dissociated mind. As main argument for this synthesis the author uses modern chaos theory that provides conceptual framework for self-organization that connect mind and brain. In this context the author also deals with the problem of consciousness and other interesting connections and mysteries of the human mind such as dreaming, hypnosis or pain experience.

FOREWORD

Purpose of this book is to present current knowledge regarding relationship between conscious and unconscious processes as it is viewed by the author in a wider interdisciplinary context. A barier between the conscious and the unconscious presents a mystery of recent knowledge and historically is linked to the term dissociation that presents the cause of the barier between conscious and unconscious psychological processes. It means that in the human mind manifest different personality states that are related to different self-reference frames exclusive to each other. For example, within this framework a mild form is splitting in perception of a close person as totally "good" or "bad" that reflects switching in self-reference as a fully accepted or fully denied person caused by high sensitivity to outside stimuli from social environment. Stressful and traumatic conditions may cause switching within a spectrum of self-reference frames related to a deficit of adaptive form of self-awareness and identity. These processes are closely related to mechanisms of consciousness, attentional mechanisms and memory processes that constitute awareness and psychological experience. In this context psychopathological processes are linked to mechanisms of pathological dissociation caused by stressful and traumatic experiences that lead to deficits in memory consolidation. These basic neurophysiological processes related to stress cause that dissociation in mental functions occurs in many psychological disorders. Within this framework dissociative identity disorder (or multiple personality disorder) can be understood as an extreme form of shame and conformity caused by stress and social pressure that determine denial of certain own feelings, ideas, patterns of behavior and resulting identity as a form of switching self-reference. These fluctuating states of consciousness and self-awareness within one human brain represent a form of personality-state-dependent information processing that is related to typical manifestation in the brain areas and networks involved in experience of the self. Following the framework of traditional psychological and psychiatric terms proposed by Janet and developed also by Freud and Jung, the recent findings suggest new connections between modern theoretical neuroscience and psychological concept of dissociated mind within the framework of self-organization and chaos theory that could enable to connect mind and brain. In this context the problem of consciousness and other interesting connections and mysteries of the human mind such as dreaming, hypnosis or pain experience could be understood within the framework that can help to find a new understanding of the brain organization and nature of conscious experience.

Chapter 1

CONSCIOUS AND SUBLIMINAL MIND

1.1. ATTENTION, PERCEPTUAL CONSCIOUSNESS AND THE SELF

According to the modern definition selective attention can be defined as selection among potential conscious contents (Baars, 1988, 2002) and specific function of attentional mechanisms is to bring different events to consciousness. This process enables global distribution of information that is located in brain regions underlying conscious processing and separated from those involved in the selection of visual objects and events (Baars, 1997, 1999, 2002).

Research of the neural correlates of consciousness (Crick and Koch, 1995) or the neural correlates of perceptual awareness repeatedly approaches to a fundamental question whether all perception is accompanied by awareness or not. Extensive evidence from behavioral studies of normal subjects as well as neurological patients show that perceptual information can be represented in the mind/brain without the subject's awareness of that information (Kanwisher, 2001). It opens the question regarding conditions that are needed for conscious experience of a neural representation. It is possible that even a strong neural representation may not be sufficient for awareness and there is behavioral evidence that perceptual awareness involves not only activation of the relevant perceptual properties but the further construction of an organized representation in which these visual properties are attributed to their sources in external objects and events (Kanwisher, 2001; Baars, 1988).

Simple examples of these cases provide ambiguous stimuli in the cases when perceptual experience alternates between two different states and lead to perceptual bistability in cases such as Necker cube (Figure 1), Rubin's face/vase or other ambiguous pictures. Similar example are experiments of binocular rivalry in which different images are projected to each eye (Kanwisher, 2001; von Helmholtz, 1962). Although the stimulus itself does not change the human observer sees only one of them, instead of seeing a mixture of the two images and their perceptual experience seems to reflect a dynamic competition between the two inputs. When for example, vertical stripes are presented to the left eye and horizontal stripes to the right eye, the viewer is likely to see not a superimposition of the two patterns (i.e. a crosshatching plaid pattern), but an alternating sequence in which only vertical stripes will be seen for one moment, and only horizontal stripes the next. Although the precise mechanisms underlying binocular rivalry are a matter of some debate it is clear that experience alternates in a bistable fashion between being dominated by the input to one eye and being dominated by the input to the other eye (Blake et al., 1998; Kanwisher, 2001).

Important phenomena that affect the contents of perceptual awareness include attention, mental imagery, and changing states of consciousness. For each of these phenomena, neural signals have been shown to be connected with perceptual awareness. As in cases described above, only simple focusing of visual attention on different aspects of an unchanging stimulus has a strong effect on the content and intensity of perceptual awareness (Rees et al., 1999). Closely following the effect of attention on subjective experience, numerous studies using single-unit recordings (Desimone and Duncan, 1995), ERPs (Luck and Girelli, 1998), and brain imaging have shown clear modulations of sensory responses by attention, even for a constant stimulus and even in primary visual cortex (Kanwisher, 2001). A rather different manipulation of perceptual awareness occurs during mental imagery, in which no stimulus is present at all and selective activation has been reported during mental imagery of motion (Goebel et al. 1998) or for face and place imagery (Kanwisher, 2001). In each of these cases, the activations during mental imagery are weaker than the corresponding stimulus activations.

Theoretical explanation of the observed phenomena proposed Desimone and Duncan (1995) in the concept of 'interactive competition'. According to this model competitive interactions across cortical areas result in domination of perceptual representations by properties of a single object. This competition can be biased by either bottom-up factors (e.g. stimulus salience) or top-down factors (e.g. endogenous attention). In either case the net result is that the various properties of an object, represented in distinct cortical regions, enhance each other and suppress the representation of competing objects. On this view, attention and awareness are global properties of the entire perceptual system that connect multiple cortical areas (Kanwisher, 2001). These principles of perceptual bistability are closely linked to dissociative states in which multistable competitive interactions and alterations in perception, emotion and identity were described. For example, in mild forms in cases of splitting in borderline personality disorder perception of a close person as totally "good" or "bad" significantly alternates (Figure 2).

These findings suggest that awareness of perceptual information requires not only a strong representation of the contents of awareness, but access to that information by other parts of the mind/brain (Baars, 1988, 2002). The limits on conscious access to perceptual information may not be immutable and for example, brain damage may disrupt neural pathways and the perceptual information represented in one neural structure is not accessed by other parts of the system (Baars, 2002). On the other hand conscious access to perceptual information may also change over time even in undamaged brains (Kanwisher, 2001). According to conscious access hypothesis consciousness might be a gateway to brain integration that enables access between otherwise separate neuronal functions (Baars, 2002). In accordance with this explanation there is evidence for a mutual dependence between consciousness and executive input and a loss of one executive interpreter's access to conscious events while another was dominant in cases of multiple personality, dissociative fugue and during hypnosis was reported (Hilgard, 1988; Putnam, 1995; Baars, 2002).

This suggests a binding between conscious contents and self functions, and similar dissociation may be found in split-brain patients where each hemisphere executive control over one side of the body, based on conscious input, is limited to half of the visual field (Gazzaniga and Sperry, 1967; Sperry, 1968). From this point of view consciousness may enable access to self functions as well (Baars, 2002).

Perceptual bi-stability as a class of phenomena in which a particular stimulus gives rise to two different interpretations therefore may reveal general principles about brain architecture (Rubin, 2003). Generally such cases results in multi-stability when each of the competing interpretations have periods of dominance and the (three or more) percepts alternate in dominance in a seemingly random manner. Multi-stable phenomena thus suggest an underlying principle of mutual exclusivity (Rubin, 2003) that is typical for perceptual consciousness as well as for dissociative phenomena. The quasistability related to different levels of interpretation process has been suggested to be connected with dynamic nonlinear chaotic processes and self-organization (Aks and Sprott, 2003) similarly as switches between dissociated behavioral states (Putnam, 1997). These findings may represent significant outlet for future research of common basis for interpretative functions in multistable perception and dissociative phenomena.

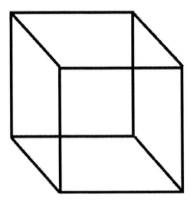

Figure 1. Necker cube.

1.2. EXPLICIT AND IMPLICIT CONSCIOUSNESS

In the above context modern study of the cognitive unconscious defined explicit and implicit perception, i.e. explicit perception means perception immediately presented to consciousness of the subject while implicit perception is not accessible for the awareness of the subject and cannot be verified immediately in the response of the subject but only indirectly by observation or measurement (Kihlstrom, 1987, 2004; Bob, 2003a). Implicit perception represents process on the unconscious level in which introspection is not possible. But also this subliminal information that remains under the limit of consciousness and is perceived unconsciously influences the organism (Kihlstrom, 1987, 2004; Bob, 2003b). A suitable method for the study of implicit perception became the subliminal stimulation (for example very short projection of an image or special forms of auditory stimulation). Libet (1979) shows that all stimuli lasting less than 500 ms with respect to a nature of the stimulus most frequently are not present in awareness of the subject. Great interest in subliminal phenomena arose from experiment performed in 1957 that led to the restriction of subliminal advertising.

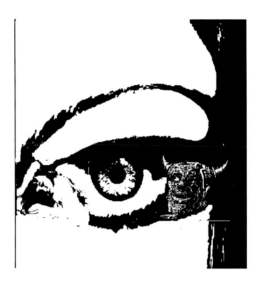

Figure 2. Because of splitting, perception of a close person as totally "good" (angel) or "bad" (demon) may significantly alternate.

During a movie presentation were projected two verbal messages: "Drink Coca-Cola" and "Eat popcorn" which led to increased popcorn consumption about 58% and Coca-Cola consumption about 18% (Wortman et al., 1992). The experiment caused controversial discussions but following findings confirmed the existence subliminal perception and information processing (Crick and Koch, 1995; Marcel, 1983; Kihlstrom, 1987; Shevrin, 2001; Bernat et al., 2001; Brazdil et al. 2001; Liddell et al., 2004) and the method of subliminal activation has been proved as a suitable instrument for the study of the dynamic and cognitive unconscious.

Further findings about subliminal processes came also from the field of neurophysiological study of the dynamic and cognitive unconscious and show complexity of information processing without awareness of the subject. It is focused mainly on the study of the dynamic unconscious connected with emotional conflict.

Experimental measurement linked to the subliminal stimulation, for example in the form of two different subliminally presented pictures enables to distinguish these different subliminally presented pictures, e.g. one which is connected to the inner conflict (for example picture of a well-known person evoking phobia) and the other which is not associated with the conflict, without any conscious activity of the patient related to these events. For example using measurement of changes in skin resistance it was shown that the neutral stimulus does not lead to any observable changes but the picture associated with the phobia results in a measurable response (Poetzl, 1960).

The phenomena of subliminal stimulation were also studied by analyzing Event Related Potentials (ERP) using P3 (also called P300) wave, which is a positive wave with latency 300 ms, after presentation of a stimulus (Brandis and Lehmann, 1986).

These studies performed on emotionally disturbed patients show that the P3 wave reflects the neurophysiological changes associated with the subliminal stimulus connected with the emotional conflict (Wong et al., 1994, 2004). Additionally, the P3 wave was able to demonstrate that the prosopagnostic patient could distinguish (albeit unconsciously) between familiar and unknown faces (Reanault et al., 1989; Eimer, 2000; Bobes et al., 2003). Other data also indicate that threshold of consciousness may change with respect to experimental conditions, for example Stross and Shevrin (1962, 1968, 1969) have shown alterations of thought contents under hypnosis in investigation of "freely evoked images" after the subliminal presentation. Their major conclusion was that hypnosis leads to heightened access to subliminal stimuli and that thought organization during hypnosis shares some common elements with thought organization during dreaming. It corresponds to similar findings when subliminally presented images were found in dreams (Fischer, 1954; Poetzl, 1960).

There are some studies, which confirm a common view that the manifestations of post hypnotic suggestion are very similar to some psychopathological phenomena (Huston et al. 1934; Vermetten and Bremner, 2004) and it is probable that psychopathological phenomena lead to a dissociated state by lowering the corresponding psychic content beneath the threshold of consciousness (Bob, 2003a).

Chapter 2

HISTORY OF DISSOCIATION AND ITS PRESENT TIMES

2.1. DISSOCIATION AND DISEASES OF MEMORY

Story of dissociation in the scientific arena began French psychologist Theódule Ribot in his book "Diseases of memory", who introduced an important concept of retrograde amnesia that was later formulated as "Ribot's Law". This principle states that brain damage has greater influence on recent than on remote memories. His work opened new era in the study of disorders of memory such as amnesia, multiple personality disorder, hysteria and other dissociative phenomena (Ellenberger, 1970). Ribot in his investigations initiated research on diseases of memory and used in this context psychological terms such as will and personality. In his thought Ribot adopted and introduced the principle of evolution and dissolution that in the field of neurology investigated famous British neurologist Hughlings Jackson (Ellenberger, 1970). This principle states that functions which appeared last in evolution and emerge late in human development, are the most fragile and are lost first. Jackson called this process "dissolution," which represents the reverse of evolution. Behavior of an individual due to dissolution is more automatic with less voluntary control and performed in a manner that is less complex than in a normal state. In addition to the loss of late-developing functions there is a discoordination among functions and exaggeration of earlier functions (Meares, 1999; Ellenberger, 1970). Ribot applied this principle to the psychopathology of memory and will. This reformulated principle states that more recent memories disappear before the earlier ones (Ribot's Law) and similarly in the case of will, where this principle expresses the findings that voluntary activities disappear before the earlier ones. This principle is a source for the later formulated theory of psychasthenia by Pierre Janet (Ellenberger, 1970) which preceded the formulation of the theory of dissociation.

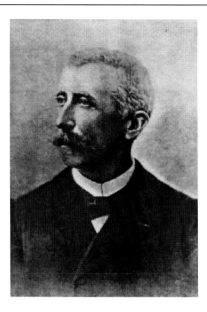

Figure 3. Theodule Ribot.

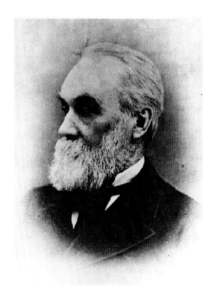

Figure 4. Hughlings Jackson.

2.2. ASSOCIATION AND DISSOCIATION

The term dissociation has its origin in the constituent parts of the term 'dis-association' which means disconnecting or lowering the strength of associative connections. Even before Janet, in the year 1845, Moreau de Tours used the term psychological dissolution (désagrégation psychologique) (van der Hart and Friedman, 1989). Analogically Hughlings Jackson (Meares, 1999) in the connection to dissolution used the term "dreamy state" which meant splitting consciousness leading to amnesia and other symptoms, such as depersonalization, derealization, hallucination or disagregation of perception. Morton Prince, one from Janet's contemporaries, used the term "co-conscious" in the sense that two consciousness are isolated from one another (Prince and Peterson, 1908; Hilgard, 1974). Max Desoir identified two main streams of mental activity as upper or lower consciousness where the lower one may emerge - for example, in hypnosis (Hilgard, 1974). F. Myers introduced the term subliminal Self which was later used also by William James (Hilgard, 1974).

Janet initially elaborated the concept of dissociation in his work Psychological Automatism (Havens 1966; Janet 1890; van der Hart and Friedman, 1989), where he sketches his notion of psychic functions and structures. He dealt with psychological phenomena often observable in hysteria, hypnosis and states of suggestion or possession. From 1889 his work was greatly influenced by his collaboration with J.M. Charcot in the Parisian hospital Salpetrière. During complete psychological automatism (van der Hart and Friedman, 1989), consciousness is totally dominated by repeating past experiences, such as in somnambulism or hysterical crises. In the case of partial automatism, only a part of the consciousness is dominated. In the case of complete or partial automatism systems of unconscious fixed ideas play an important role and repress conscious control and perception. They may emerge in many forms of psychopathological or somatoform symptoms, for example paroxysm, which may be understood as a representation of psychological trauma when a fixed idea is transformed into hallucinations and body movements (van der Hart and Friedman, 1989). Fixed ideas are presented in the form of dreams and dissociative episodes (e.g. hysterical attacks) or during hypnosis as a secondary consciousness. A characteristic feature of these states is a lowering of the mental level (abaissement du niveau mental), which is manifested by increased dissociation and mental depression connected to the reduction of psychological tension. According to C.G. Jung due to dissociation psychic entities are created and associated with certain contents of memory, patterns of behavior, and emotional charges. Jung called these entities "psychic complexes". A complex always has its own autonomy and behaves as a split part of the psyche. When a complex is evoked into the consciousness, its physiological or pathological influence depends on a degree of its autonomy. In the case of pathological influence the complex leads to a lowered mental level (Janet, 1890; van der Hart and Friedman 1989). As Janet suggested, the fundamental causes of the etiology of pathological complexes are mainly traumatic events, which produce traumatic memories. Complexes thus generate alternate fields of the psyche, and it is possible, by means of these complexes, to explain extreme cases of dissociation which occur in multiple personality disorder (Bob, 2004). Complexes represent organized collections of ideas, emotions, impulses, and memories with a common emotional tone which have been excluded either partly or entirely from consciousness but continue to influence a person's thoughts, emotions, and behavior (Colman, 2003). Complexes are pathologically disintegrated due to abnormal intensive affect compensated by neural inhibition. Failure of this inhibition manifests itself as a continuum of pathological dissociation from mild forms, such as repression, to serious forms, such as splitting or word salad. Inhibited negative emotion is dissociated from the consciousness and it implicates the problem of unconscious emotions which in serious states of dissociation lead to phenomenological fragmentation of the Self to multiple Selves (Lambie and Marcel, 2002, 2004; Dalgleish and Power, 2004).

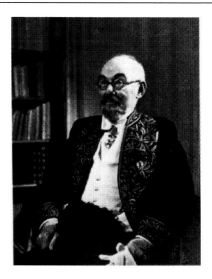

Figure 5. Pierre Janet.

2.3. DISSOCIATION AND REPRESSION

Similarly but later than Janet, Sigmund Freud and Joseph Breuer even considered double consciousness in "Studies in hysteria" (Breuer and Freud, 1895). Breuer and Freud conceptualized pathological conditions observed in conversion phenomena as a consequence of repression and according to them "dissociated states" are elicited by the repression of the libido energy. At the beginning of psychoanalysis Freud began his project on scientific psychopathology with the purpose to find brain mechanisms related to cognitive functions that constitute normal and abnormal mental processes (Ellenberger, 1970; Rofe, 2008). Freud elaborated the theory of the unconscious based on apriori postulate that unconscious mind is biological in nature and proposed conceptual identity connecting mind and brain within his neurological theory. His collaboration with Joseph Breuer uncovered new development in psychology and provided new conceptual framework for understanding of the mind-body problem in which mental and somatic factors are closely connected and understood as different aspects of a unity (Ellenberger, 1970; Breuer and Freud, 1895; Briquet, 1859, Mace, 1992).

Following development suggests that both concepts dissociation and repression are significantly different in their approach to psychotherapy, which has historical roots in the term abreaction introduced by Joseph Breuer. As historical data show, first literary documented utilization of this method has been described by Janet in his patient Lucie in 1886 (Janet, 1886; Ellenberger, 1970) and later used and defined this method Joseph Breuer in his famous patient Anna (Breuer and Freud, 1895). According to definition of the American Psychiatric Association abreaction is defined as: "…an emotional release or discharge after recalling a painful experience that has been repressed because it was consciously intolerable. A therapeutic effect sometimes occurs through partial discharge or de-sensitization of the painful emotions and increased insight. (American Psychiatric Association, 1980, p. 1)". This definition embodies historical controversy between French school of dissociation and later studies by Joseph Breuer and Sigmund Freud, who for the understanding of abreactive process utilized the concept of repression in their "Studies of Hysteria" (Breuer and Freud, 1895) and understood abreaction as a discharge of repressed energy linked to traumatic memory.

As later development showed, definition of a nature of abreactive experience has key consequences for understanding of therapeutic process as integration of dissociative state ("double conscience") or on the contrary as discharge of repressed energy linked to traumatic memory. Further research and clinical practice suggest that repeated abreactions without integration of dissociated state often has malignant effect without any improvement of the patient state and lead to strengthening intrusive symptoms (van der Hart and Brown, 1992). Integrative view of abreactive process suggested Putnam (1989), who for the purpose of therapeutically controlled abreactions emphasized the importance of reliving of the traumatic experience as well as the discharge of related affects and integration of traumatic material into conscious awareness during and after the abreactive experience. Also other authors warned against activation of traumatic memories during the abreaction without an appropriate cognitive framework which is necessary for adequate defenses or coping skills and recommended that emotions should be expressed in a planned, safer and controlled manner (Brown and Fromm, 1986; Horowitz, 1986; Braun, 1986; Ross, 1989).

According to recent clinical evidence abreaction represents useful clinical instrument for the treatment of certain dissociation related disturbances. This evidence also suggests that the expression and discharge of an affect during the revivification of traumatic memories (useful also under hypnosis) must enable re-integration of dissociated parts of the traumatic memory and assimilate the traumatic event into the whole of the personality (van der Hart and Brown, 1992; Putnam 1992; Watkins and Watkins, 2000).

Later development in the theory of dissociation after First World War continued only in the field of psychoanalysis and Janet's work was almost ignored. This great interest in psychoanalysis after the First World War caused that French roots of psychoanalysis in Freud's studies in Salpetrière in 1885-86 (in J.M. Charcot) almost fall into oblivion (Ellenberger, 1970; Haule, 1984).

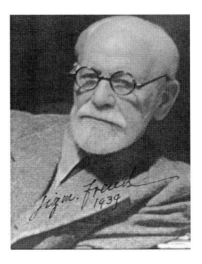

Figure 6. Sigmund Freud.

2.4. HILGARD'S NEODISSOCIATION THEORY

Some new interest in the theory of dissociation appeared after the Second World War along with a restoration of interest in the study of hypnosis. Ernest R. Hilgard who continued in Janet's tradition in his neodissociation theory sketched in the work "Toward a Neodissociation Theory: Multiple Cognitive Controls in Human Functioning" (Hilgard, 1974) and comprehensively described in his book (Hilgard, 1986) returned to and significantly developed Janet's concept for understanding hypnosis.

According to Hilgard, secondary dissociated consciousness is characterized by a 'hidden observer' which has the characteristics of a central stream of consciousness towards which information from many secondary streams or personalities converges. A similar phenomenon was described as the 'internal self-helper' in multiple personality disorder (Lynn et al. 1994; Hilgard 1986). Several authors point to clinical findings that experiences under hypnosis support the view that something similar to multiple personality may also be present in people who have not been given this diagnosis (Gabel, 1989; Saley, 1988).

These findings suggest that human psychic system may be understood as an ordered system of complexes with self-function related to structured mental representations and neuronal assemblies with many associated connections which are differentiated by the strength of the synaptic connections between them. The complex which most often dominates was called the ego complex by Jung, and in multiple personality it corresponds to the primary personality. Other personalities, called secondary, correspond to the other complexes. Multiple personality thus may be considered as a structural model of the dissociated human personality. 'The hidden observer' corresponds to some of the empirical findings that led Jung to introduce the term the 'Self'. In this context, dreams may be considered as a vehicle for disseminating information among the dissociated elements of the human personality (Gabel, 1989; Saley, 1988). These are some of the key features of neo-dissociation theory.

These ideas are supported by research findings of hypnotic dissociated consciousness, for example in relation to hypnotic analgesia, such as the phenomenon of automatic writing, whilst the attention of the subject under investigation was taken up by a distracting activity. During these experiments, the subject was pricked with a needle into the hypnotically anaesthetized left-hand. The subject's right hand wrote the sentence 'you hurt me' even though the hypnotized subject denied any awareness of pain (Hilgard, 1986). Automatic writing under hypnosis was an experimental technique that Janet had already used to obtain information which was inaccessible to the subject consciousness and was stored in implicit memory.

In further experiments with hypnotic analgesia the process of evoking painful memories detected by the 'hidden observer'was also investigated. These clinical studies support the view that information about pain is registered and stored during hypnotic analgesia, as Hilgard's experiments demonstrated. Experiments undertaken in Canada suggest that the 'hidden observer' is not an experimental artifact (Hilgard, 1986). Together these findings indicate that dissociative processes must be seen as a clinical reality, although the concept of the 'hidden observer' as a cognitive phenomenon of implicit knowledge suggests that dissociation between pain and consciousness is not complete.

2.5. HYPNOSIS AND SUBLIMINAL INFORMATION PROCESSING

Further research on pain sensation in hypnosis shows that information about pain, due to cognitive modulation leading to analgesia or anesthesia, is either not accessible or less accessible to the conscious mind. According to some findings, it may be processed at a subliminal level and memory of it may be recalled during hypnosis (Chertok, Michaux, and Droin, 1977; Nogrady et al., 1983; Wolfe and Millet, 1960; Hilgard, 1986). Hilgard (1986) called this subliminal level "the hidden observer". Typical example of Hilgard's experiment is following: A subject was told that his left hand would feel no pain when plunged into a bucket of ice-cold water. Under hypnosis, the subject confirmed that he felt no pain. Then the subject was asked to allow his right hand to engage in some "automatic writing" (that is, to let the hand write anything it wanted). "It is freezing", wrote the hand, "it hurts" and then: "Take my hand out." The "hidden observer" manifests as a dissociated conscious state that represents cognitive dimension divided from subject awareness. In some other cases a patient under hypnosis (his "hidden observer") remembered experienced pain during surgery and described the course of an operation performed under complete anesthesia. In these cases, the hidden observer described pain experience as independent witness (Chertok, Michaux, and Droin, 1977; Nogrady et al., 1983; Wolfe and Millet, 1960). This phenomenon was reported also by Levinson (1967) and Cheek (1959, 1964, 1966) in cases when anesthesia was induced pharmacologically. Although the evidence of the hidden observer is controversial (Lynn et al., 1994; Kirsch and Lynn, 1998), these findings increased interest in study of perceiving pain without conscious experience. Similar phenomena occurred in patients after prefrontal lobectomy and led to definition of two levels of pain. The first level is related to pain experience called "suffering pain" and the second represents informational dimension called "sensory pain" that may be perceived "unconsciously" (Chertok, Michaux, and Droin, 1977; Melzack and Cassey, 1968). These definitions implicate two levels in processing of nociceptive stimuli, the first, accessible to subject awareness and the second, dissociated from subject consciousness that exists on the subliminal level. The concept of sensory pain per se is in accordance with extensive evidence from behavioral studies of normal subjects as well as neurological patients which show that perceptual information can be represented in the mind and brain without the subject's awareness of that information (Fernandez-Duque, 2003; Mericle et al., 2001; Kihlstrom, 2004; Shevrin, 2001; Smith and Bulman-Fleming, 2004). These data suggest a subliminal level of consciousness consistently with the concept of attentional filtering mechanism that discriminates among mental events and ignores a part of this perceptual information and intentional attitudes that influence other psychological processes outside of conscious awareness (Gawronski, Hofmann, and Wilbur, 2006; Lesley, 2006; Toates, 2006; Pestana, 2006; Natsoulas, 2006).

Studies in hypnosis also show that a lowering of the threshold of consciousness leads not only to the manifestation of dissociated components of the personality but also to the discovery of an integrative entity called the 'hidden observer', which in multiple personality operates as an internal self-helper that seems to be aware of other sub-personalities, even though these subpersonalities are completely dissociated from each other. One example might be the case in which a patient, who had undergone an operation under anaesthetic, was unable consciously to recall the procedure but under hypnosis the 'hidden observer' could give an account of the operation and could describe the pain, but as if it was experienced by somebody else (Hilgard, 1986). This phenomenon, in which, under hypnosis, the 'hidden observer' could describe events occurring when that person was previously under anaesthesia, was also confirmed by Levinson (1967) and by Cheek (1959, 1966). It may be the case that the 'hidden observer' may provide an explanation for phenomena such as 'Near Death' and 'Out of Body' experiences. In addition, Lynn et al. (1994) suggest that the 'hidden observer' in hypnosis or hypnotic dreams may be able to provide information about personal experiences that is otherwise unavailable to conscious recall, including traumatic events such as physical or sexual abuse. These authors also found evidence of the 'hidden observer' in 80% of nonhypnotized subjects who were in a relaxed state. It is possible that mystical experiences may represent a moment of manifestation of the unconscious 'counterpart' or 'hidden observer' and can be explained in these terms.

2.5. COMPLEXES AND DISCRETE BEHAVIORAL STATES

Jung's complex theory in many of its aspects corresponds to modern formulation of discrete behavioral states by Frank Putnam (1997) who's work presents very significant contribution to the history dissociation. According to Putnam discrete behavioral states provide alternative perspective for the understanding of dissociation. The term discrete behavioral states originates from the study of infant mental states. Infant behavioral states can be defined by a set of observable continuous and dichotomous variables. The number of infant states and their levels of interconnection increase with development and are responsible for the infant's growing behavioral repertoire. Healthy children are born with basic set of behavioral states. Fundamental features of a system of discrete states of consciousness are different state dependent behaviors in response to the same stimulus.

In adults, this type of differential responsiveness is most apparent in such disorders as bipolar illness or multiple personality disorder (Putnam, 1997). State defining variables may be continuous or dichotomous and define behavioral state space. It means that individual behavioral states existing within larger multidimensional framework or space, defined by a chosen set of variables, occupy discrete volumes of the state space. An individual's behavior traverses the state space in a series of discontinuous jumps or switches from one state to another (Putnam, 1997). The state space may be vast but individual regularly occupies those regions in which one has created stable discrete states (Putnam, 1997). The discrete states as transitory behavioral structures are linked together by directional pathways forming behavioral architecture that defines an individual's personality. Transition between behavioral states is manifested as "switch" that represents abrupt change in the values of the constellation of state defining variables, for example transition from waking to sleeping or in bipolar illness from mania to depression (Putnam, 1997). Model of discrete behavioral states defines "pathological dissociation" as a trauma induced discrete behavioral states that are widely separated in multidimensional state space from normal states of consciousness and it corresponds to conventional definition, which emphasize the separation or segregation of specific ideas or affects from normal mental phenomena (Putnam, 1997; Kaplan and Sadock,

1991). When two types of states are significantly different, then the states are separated by a wide gap in state space that determines pathological dissociative states. Observable differences between two discrete states are not a simple function of moving up or down. Putnam suggested that these processes could be related to nonlinear dynamic features connected to chaos (Putnam, 1997). In this context, for example Wolff (1987) highlights differential responsiveness as an example of the nonlinearity of input-output relation in different states of consciousness and conceptualizes the relevance of nonlinear dynamic systems theory to discrete behavioral states where switches between behavioral states constitute nonlinear transitions. Further recent studies give stronger evidence that rapid shifts in mood and behavior could be related to nonlinear dynamic processes (Putnam, 1997; Gottschalk et al. 1995).

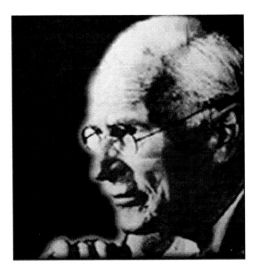

Figure 7. Carl G. Jung.

2.6. DISSOCIATION AND STATE DEPENDENT LEARNING

In the context of discrete behavioral states, important concept in the history of dissociation presents the theory of state dependent learning. The basic principle of the state dependent learning is that something what was learned in one neuropsychophysiological state is best recalled in the same state (Brown, 1984). Explanation of this phenomenon is often based on experiments with animals which show that an experimental animal under influence of a drug, store memory information in a neural state that is not possible to recall without the drug. It could be explained within the concept of neural plasticity in a way that during influence of a drug new neuronal connections are created and that the drug is necessary for their reactivation because the drug is included in the memory process and influences neuronal excitability and sensitivity that must be renewed for recall of the memory contents.

In the above context, experiments in humans confirm that there is a relationship between difficulty of the task and its recall, and that the type of the task influences the result (Brown, 1984). Tasks more complicated have higher effect of state dependent learning than simple motor tasks. This effect was also shown in stress situations or in emotional states (Henry et al., 1973; Pearce et al., 1990) and in sleep and circadian rhytmicity (Holloway, 1978). Similarly, research of postictal states confirmed that state dependent learning is not a result of the drug influence but presents an important brain property (Overton, 1978). Important finding is also an effect of state dependent learning as a consequence of changes in mood (Bower, 1981) reported also in cases of maniodepresive states induced by dextroamphetamin application (Henry et al., 1973). Similar influence of emotional states was also confirmed using hypnosis (Brown, 1984; Bower, 1981). Within this context state dependent learning supports the view that dissociation is related to selective specialization of cognitive functions due to changes in environment and situations in life.

2.7. DISSOCIATION AND NEURAL NETWORK MODELS

The state dependent learning also motivated development of formalized models of dissociation using neural network. First proposed model of a neural network suitable for the study of dissociative processes was suggested by Bower (Bower, 1981; Butler et al., 1996). In this model memory is saved in single elements of the network. The memory content may be excited when its corresponding memory element is activated upon reaching a threshold. In the network there are elements with excitation influences on memory contents and also elements that inhibit them, and Bower assumed that dissociative disorders can be related to neurobiological mechanisms of the state dependent learning (Yates and Nasby, 1993).

Later conceptual model used the principle of the parallel operation of two or more information processors (Li and Spiegel, 1992). In dissociation these processor neural systems are disintegrated (Li and Spiegel, 1992). This conceptualizes model of neural networks with parallel distributed memory in the space of the network (Butler et al. 1996; Li and Spiegel 1992; Mc Clelland and Rumelhart 1986). This neural network model seems to be able to explain a wider class of dissociative processes, such as the course of posthypnotic amnesia. In this context Parallel Distributed Processing (PDP) presents a model for the microstructure of cognition (Mc Clelland and Rumelhart 1986). Activities of many neurons are described as configurations or neural patterns and their psychological correlates present mental representations (Butler et al. 1996; Li and Spiegel, 1992; Mc Clelland and Rumelhart, 1986). In this description the neural network state is described by the superposition of neuronal patterns. Potential neural patterns and configurations in their "superposition" are in "prespace", which might be attributed to psychic space and the active neural patterns are selected from this superposition (Butler et al. 1996; Li and Spiegel, 1992; Mc Clelland and Rumelhart, 1986).

2.8. DISSOCIATION, BRAIN COMPLEXITY AND CHAOS

Because dissociation represents an inability to integrate some psychic contents, such as from memory into the consciousness (Bernstein and Putnam, 1986; Kruger and Mace, 2002) the disintegration represents the problem rather than the competition of these subsystems (Li and Spiegel, 1992). In this context, dissociative states present mental representations, which are inaccessible to dominant interpreter's access that could be in principle related to dominant ego-complex, i.e. dominant consciousness or dominant subpersonality in multiple personality disorder. In accordance with Baars' (2002) conscious access hypothesis it has not access to certain contents of memory, consciousness or identity that present dissociated part of the mind. From this inaccessibility and other aspects of dissociative states may be inferred that between the brain states representing dissociated mental representations an antagonistic competitive relationship occurs. As suggested above these states can be modeled using the concept of parallel distributed processing in neural networks (Butler et al. 1996; Li and Spiegel, 1992; Mc Clelland and Rumelhart, 1986). Many activity configurations in parallel distributed processing networks are represented as points in an N-dimensional plane, where N represents number of neurons in the network. In a most simple case we can propose the model of two neurons and all their possible activities defined by synaptic strength that can be represented by two axes. The third axis represents the probability of a given configuration. This produces a three-dimensional plan (landscape) and "peaks" in this plane represent favored activity states. Isolated peaks in this plane represent dissociated states (Li and Spiegel, 1992). All configurations in the N-dimensional plane represent a multistable dynamic system, which is changed over time with each new input. This PDP model may be used for the modeling of some pathological states, for example functional amnesia, multiple personality disorder and post-traumatic stress disorder (Butler et al. 1996; Li and Spiegel, 1992; Mc Clelland and Rumelhart, 1986; Bob, 2003b).

In this context, dissociation on neurophysiological level in principle could be described using the concept of brain complexity. Generally, the complexity of the system means simply its composition from simple units or its dimensionality and tends to evolve over time (Coveney and Highfield, 1996). Structures, which have a higher number of dimensions, are generally viewed as more complex. In the case of neural networks or an electroencephalogram this means that there is competition among oscillating neuronal cell assemblies (neural configurations). Complexity is, for example, higher during divergent (creative) thinking than during convergent thinking (analytical thought) (Mölle et al., 1996), which leads to suppression of the competition among neural assemblies. Also, people with higher intelligence have higher EEG complexity (Lutzenberger et al., 1992). Complexity and competition among neural cell assemblies can be represented by a number of simultaneously active neuronal assemblies involved in performing of a task. For example, during convergent analytical thought all information irrelevant for solving the problem is reduced and at the same time the number of competitive neural assemblies is reduced and the complexity decreases. Higher competition during creative thinking leads to the establishment of new associations among neural representations of mental states (Mölle et al., 1996). These findings implicate transient periods of high complexity of the EEG during activity of independent areas that enables fast parallel information processing which runs in a distributed mode. It means that numerous processes from sensory and cognitive channels are executed simultaneously and this desynchronized neural state may be related to active information processing in the cortex (Tirsch et al., 2004). Competition among cortical neural cell assemblies which excite one another and are unable to agree on a common frequency of oscillations (Freeman, 1991) thus may be used as appropriate neurophysiological equivalent to dissociated and disintegrated competitive mental states in PDP model (Bob, 2003b). When the associated strength in these newly activated ranges of the neural network is low, it leads to strong competition among the neural assemblies (Freeman, 1991), and dissociated mental representations (Bob, 2003b). In parallel distributed processing model these dissociated states with low associated strength are represented by isolated "peaks" (Mc Clelland and Rumelhart, 1986; Li and Spiegel, 1992; Butler et al., 1996).

2.9. DISSOCIATION AND EPILEPTIFORM ACTIVITY

Typical changes in complexity related to dissociation could be in principle related to epileptiform abnormalities and epileptic EEG activity, repeatedly found in dissociated patients (Putnam, 1997; Teicher et al., 2003).

A clear distinction of the relationship between epileptic and epileptiform discharges shows relationship between ictal and interictal symptomatology. While epilepsy is defined as a chronic condition characterized by spontaneous, recurrent seizures and seizure is defined as a clinical event associated with a transient, hypersynchronous neuronal discharge (epileptic is a descriptive term used to denote the presence of epilepsy), epileptiform discharges is an interpretive term used in electroencephalography that applies to distinctive waves or complexes distinguishable from the background activity, which resemble the waveforms recorded in a proportion of human subjects suffering from an epileptic disorder (Chatrian et al., 1974). Epileptiform patterns include spike and sharp waves, alone or accompanied by slow waves, occurring singly or in bursts lasting at most a few seconds. The term epileptiform typically refers to interictal paroxysmal activity and not to the EEG activity seen during an actual seizure, which is called an electrographic seizure (Chatrian et al., 1974).

In this terminological context recent data indicate that traumatic stress and dissociation might be significantly related to epileptiform activity (Putnam, 1997; Teicher et al. 2003). Because epileptiform and epileptic activity represents typical example of chaos in neural organization (Korn and Faure, 2003; Tirsch et al., 2004) and dissociation is hypothetically attributed to neural chaotic organization it is needed to more comprehensively consider the data that have documented a relationship between dissociation and epileptic activity. The epilepsy/temporal lobe dysfunction model of dissociation was for the first time proposed by Charcot in 1892 (Putnam, 1997). This concept for explanation of neurobiological basis of dissociation is related to clinical data that prevalence of seizure disorders is much higher in multiple personality disorder patients (Mesulam, 1981; Schenk and Bear, 1981; Benson, 1986; Perrine, 1991; Putnam, 1997). On the other hand dissociation-like symptoms such as depersonalization, fugues, amnesias and autoscopy (seeing an externalized image of oneself) are sometimes reported ictally and periictally, by seizure patients (Putnam, 1997). Kindling as a neurobiological mechanism (Goddard et al. 1969) can potentially explain how epileptic-like phenomena might arise from repeated trauma (Post et al. 1995; Putnam, 1997; Teicher et al. 2003). The kindling related to traumatic stress similarly as experimental kindling likely is caused by progressively increasing response of groups of neurons due to repetitive subthreshold stimulation that may later lead to epileptic activity. It corresponds to clinical data that raise the possibility that temporal lobe abnormalities may play a role in pathological dissociation (Putnam, 1997). Typical EEG abnormalities found in traumatized and dissociated patients often involve temporal or frontal slow wave activity and also may involve frontotemporal spikes or sharp waves predominantly in the left hemisphere (Putnam, 1997; Teicher et al. 2003).

Recent studies (Putnam, 1997; Ito et al. 1993; Teicher et al. 1993, 2003) have found frequent and unusual EEG abnormalities in victims of child abuse and also several imaging studies describe hippocampal abnormalities in trauma patients (Bremner et al. 1995; Putnam 1997; Bremner, 2006; Teicher et al. 2003, 2006). Although dissociative disorders cannot be generally explained on the basis of neurological dysfunction, contemporary data supports the suggestive evidence that temporal lobe seizure activity can produce dissociative syndrome, which is similar to that observed in functional cases (Spiegel, 1991). From these findings it may be inferred that temporal lobe epileptic activity is important in the generation of dissociative symptoms without neurological focal lesion (Spiegel, 1991). It is in accordance with evidence linking dissociative symptoms to the temporal lobe activity and corresponds to clinical data that the dissociative symptoms in temporal lobe epileptics occur during interictal periods and not during the ictal state (Spiegel, 1991). Epileptic activity in interictal periods in temporal lobe epileptics also may produce characteristic symptoms called complex partial seizure-like symptoms that appear as intrusions into the normal state of consciousness in the form of cognitive, psychosensory or affective symptoms (Roberts, 1993; Roberts et al. 1990; Silberman et al. 1985; Hines et al. 1995). Many of these symptoms were already defined by Hughlings Jackson in his classical studies (Roberts et al. 1990; Dreifuss, 1981; Roberts et al. 1992). Modern findings support the view that these symptoms have, similarly as dissociation (Bernstein and Putnam, 1986), in the general population a continuous character (Roberts et al. 1990, 1992). The continuum of complex partial seizure-like symptoms begins in healthy state without the symptoms via transitional pathological states until the symptoms of complex partial epilepsy with all typical manifestations. Between these opposites a broad spectrum of different clinical dysfunctions with good response to anticonvulsant drugs occurs. It concerns most often affective diseases or atypical psychoses with characteristic manifestations of the symptoms of temporal lobe epilepsy in nonepileptic conditions and are called Epilepsy Spectrum Disorders (Roberts et al. 1992, 1999; Hines et al. 1995; Jampala et al. 1992). According to some findings (Roberts, 1993, Bob et al. 2005, 2006a) these symptoms are in close relationship to increased sensitivity on parental influence and dissociative tendency due to traumatic or aversive events most often in connection to child abuse. Two main characteristic features of these patients are enhanced dissociative capacity and abnormal electrophysiological activity (Roberts, 1993; Hines et al. 1995) although it must not be present in scalp EEG (Walker et al., 2002).

Repeated stressful events also may determine sensitization leading to an increase in responsiveness to stress stimuli resulting to significantly increased vulnerability to stressors that have more lasting consequences with kindling-like progression (Post et al., 1995; Post and Weiss, 1998; Kraus, 2000). The kindling-model of stress-related sensitization (Post et al., 1995) seems to be in agreement with suggestive evidence that stress may influence significantly increased occurrence of EEG abnormalities that have been reported in significantly traumatized patients mainly in the frontotemporal region, which consisted of spikes, sharp waves, or paroxysmal slowing, predominantly in the left hemisphere (Teicher et al., 1993, 2003, 2006; Putnam, 1997; Ito et al., 1993). Stress-related sensitization has been proposed to cause changes in GABA postsynaptic receptors that may lead to overstimulation of neurons mainly in the limbic system, resulting in limbic system irritability manifesting as markedly increased prevalence of symptoms suggestive of temporal lobe epilepsy (Teicher et al., 2003, 2006; Post et al., 1995; Bob, 2007c). Recent data strongly suggest that traumatic stress may determine limbic irritability and temporal-limbic seizure-like activity (Teicher et al., 2003, 2006; Spigelman et al., 2002; Bob et al., 2005, 2007a) and close link between limbic irritability and defects in cerebellar vermis has been reported (Teicher et al., 2003, 2006; Anderson et al., 2002).

These findings suggest that cognitive and emotional dysregulation related to traumatic stress likely is linked to defective inhibitory functions that may also lead to temporo-limbic seizure-like activity. This epileptic-like process may emerge in the form of symptoms similar to ictal temporal lobe epilepsy such as somatic, sensory, behavioral and memory symptoms that may occur also in nonepileptic conditions (Teicher et al., 2003, 2006; Silberman et al., 1985; Roberts et al., 1992; Hines et al., 1993; Bob, 2004b, 2007c).

There were also described clinical cases of EEG abnormalities related to presence of dissociative symptomes, several dissociative syndromes (including the patients with multiple personality) and also identity shift in temporal lobe epilepsy (Schenk and Bear, 1981; Mesulam, 1981; Coons et al. 1982; Benson et al. 1986; Spiegel, 1991; Ahern et al. 1993; Hersh et al. 2002). For example Ahern et al. (1993) examined the relationship of "multiple personality disorder" in two patients with temporolimbic epilepsy. Both patients had presented with different "personalities" in a characteristic temporal relationship to their seizures. These "different personalities" were known by the patient's families to manifest themselves in the postictal period.

In this context dissociative states are also present during the so-called altered states of consciousness such as possession, out of body experiences, near death experiences (Putnam, 1989) and several studies reported epileptic activity related to religious experiences (Saver and Rabin, 1997) or out of body experiences (Blanke et al., 2002).

Dissociation is also traditionally connected to inner conflict and several clinical studies indicate that activation of inner conflict during stressful interview may produce seizure activity in epileptics (Stevens, 1959, Faber et al., 1996) or activates burst waves in closed eyes in normal healthy people (Berkhout et al., 1969). There are also studies describing subcortical epileptiform activity during intensive emotional and psychopathological states (Faber and Vladyka, 1987; Heath, 1962, 1975; Groethuysen et al., 1957; Monroe, 1978, 1982; Stevens, 1999; Alvarez, 2001).

2.10. Dissociative Seizures and Psychosomatic Symptoms

Important data regarding relationship between dissociation and epilepsy present also dissociative seizures also called psychogenic nonepileptic seizures that are in DSM IV and ICD 10 diagnosed as dissociative disorders. Main etiological factor is probably dissociative process which may lead to conversion into somatic symptoms. This diagnostic classification of psychogenic nonepileptic seizures is due to growing evidence that these patients have a great deal of dissociative symptoms (Kuyk et al., 1999; Brown and Trimble, 2000). Prevalency of these pseudoseizures is not accurately known but probably it is 10-25% of all the patients visiting epileptologist specialists (Kuyk et al., 1999). Coexisting pseudoseizures and epilepsy have about 12-36% (Kuyk et al., 1999) and according to more recent data about 9-50% of all the visiting patients (Brown and Trimble, 2000). In epileptologist practice pseudoseizures and epilepsy are differentiated by finding of epileptic discharges on scalp EEG although also in patients with dissociative seizures subcortical epileptic discharges in limbic structures probably occur (Wieser, 1979).

This situation when subtle and on scalp EEG invisible seizures hardly differentiable from "true" epileptic seizures may be produced by dissociation suggests interesting possibility to understand other somatoform manifestations of dissociation in the so-called conversion disorders due to epileptiform activity which is able to produce a wide spectrum of somatic (as well as psychopathological) symptoms. Historically are these pathological manifestations associated with the term hysteria described by Pierre Janet, Joseph Breuer and Sigmund Freud in which mental and somatic factors are closely connected and understood as different aspects of a unity (Ellenberger, 1970). These pathological conditions were later re-defined by Janet as a consequence of dissociative reactions, which can lead to psychopathological as well as somatoform symptoms. Epileptic discharges as well are able to produce a wide range of psychopathological symptoms such as depression, psychosis, anxiety and other (Mace, 1993; Roberts et al., 1992) as well as a wide spectrum of somatic manifestations mainly due to autonomic symptoms of epileptic seizures (Cerullo et al., 1998; Baumgartner et al., 2001; Devinsky, 2004). Autonomic symptoms accompany other seizure symptoms or may occur as sole or predominant seizure manifestation due to an activation of the central autonomic network. Spectrum of autonomic seizure manifestations is wide ranging and can be divided into cardiovascular changes, respiratory manifestations, gastrointestinal symptoms, cutaneous manifestations, pupillary symptoms, genital and sexual manifestations as well as urinary symptoms etc. Autonomic symptoms may be also lateralized as a consequence of a hemispheric-specific representation of the central autonomic network. It is known that these symptoms may occur similarly as various motor seizures also in non-epileptic conditions and represent difficult problem for differential diagnostics (Baumgartner et al., 2001; Freeman and Schachter, 1995; Reeves, 1997). These data suggest close relationship between several somatoform dissociative states and the non-convulsive epileptic activity in autonomic nervous system, mainly in non-epileptic conditions, when subcortical epileptic discharges related to dissociative processes may produce a wide spectrum of autonomic somatoform symptoms. Known symptoms of epileptic activity linked to sensory, sensitive and motor manifestations of seizures (Dreifus, 1981; Barry et al., 1985; Ghosh, Mohanty and Prabhakar, 2001) might explain how non-convulsive epileptic activity as a consequence of dissociation may produce also other forms of somatoform dissociative symptoms such as alterations in sensation of pain (analgesia, kinesthetic anesthesia), painful symptoms, perception alterations, motor inhibition or loss of motor control, psychogenic blindness etc., which occur in conversion and somatoform disorders. These findings are important with respect to known interactions between mental state and autonomic activation. Mental stress for example influences blood pressure, formation of ulcers, esophageal motility or cardiac arrhythmias in the absence of cardiovascular predisposing factors. This relationship when mental state influences specific patterns of autonomic activation principally coordinated by cortical components of the limbic network may be important for future research which may well determine that these parts of the brain provide potential anatomical substrate for psychosomatic diseases such as essential hypertension and certain types of heart diseases (Mesulam, 1999).

2.11. FORCED NORMALIZATION AS A MODEL OF RELATIONSHIP BETWEEN PSYCHOPATHOLOGY AND SEIZURES

In this context interesting model for understanding the relationship between psychic and somatoform dissociative symptoms presents the process called forced normalization. In these pathological conditions epileptic activity– similarly as in dissociative state– may produce seizures and psychopathological symptoms.

The relationship between seizures and psychopathology is historically linked to biological antagonism between epilepsy and psychosis that was for the first time investigated by a Hungarian physician László von Meduna (Meduna, 1934; Wolf and Trimble, 1985; Krishnamoorthy et al., 2002). After graduation Meduna was interested in brain anatomy and in the year 1927 began his psychiatric research. At the time of his most important works he was leading physician in Royal Asylum in Budapest. There he dealt with experimental epilepsy and his findings confirmed that the relationship between epileptic paroxysms and psychotic manifestations is not only random (Wolf and Trimble, 1985; Krishnamoorthy et al. 2002). Meduna followed the study by Steiner and Strauss (Wolf and Trimble, 1985) who investigated 6000 schizophrenic patients and found typical epileptic paroxysms in these cases very rare. In his work from 1935 Meduna introduced the study of 176 patients from which 95 were epileptics and had at the same time also psychotic symptoms (Meduna, 1935). In this study Meduna confirmed that next to the antagonism may be also combination between epilepsy and psychosis. In his practical therapy he used convulsive drugs, for example camphor or penetrazol, for the treatment of schizophrenia. These drugs often may cause convulsions and lowering of schizophrenic symptoms (Wolf and Trimble, 1985).

Discussions following Meduna's works initiated the development of convulsive therapy in psychiatry but the relationship between epilepsy and psychosis was neglected for a time. Its investigation was renewed in 1950s when Heinrich Landolt, director of Swiss asylum for epileptics in Zürich, by means of electroencephalographical methods reported his findings on forced normalization (Wolf and Trimble, 1985; Landolt, 1953). Landolt introduced the term forced normalization for the reaction of the organism, which represents the defense of the brain against epileptic discharges (Wolf and Trimble, 1985). According to his findings this reaction may begin spontaneously or as a consequence of antiepileptic medication. First of all Landolt studied forced normalization in patients with temporal lobe epilepsy and later also in patients with focal cortical epileptic seizures. In 1954 he used succinimid medication in patients with generalized epilepsy of the type petit mal and in twilight states that represent qualitative changes of mental state dissociated from normal state of consciousness similar to schizophrenic symptoms.

Effects of forced normalization were also reported in cases of neurosurgical treatment focused on inactivation of the epileptic focus (Mace and Trimble, 1991; Blumer et al. 1998). It was suggested that the effects might explain kindling in mesolimbic dopaminergic system that has a relationship of reciprocity with regard to similar EEG activity in temporal neocortex in patients with temporal lobe epilepsy (Pakalnis et al. 1988).

Similar relationship of reciprocity was found also between epilepsy and depression (Jobe et al. 1999; Kanner and Balabanov, 2002; Chaplin et al. 1990; Trimble, 1996). Historical roots of this problem are also connected to the term forced normalization and contemporary is thought that people with epilepsy exhibit a higher incidence of depression compared to people in general population (Jobe et al. 1999; Kanner and Balabanov, 2002). In this context several sources show that there is a relationship between seizures and affective disorders (Jobe et al. 1999; Kanner and Balabanov, 2002). First reason is that electroconvulsive therapy has a high degree of efficacy in the treatment of depression as well as in the treatment of manic states and similarly it is also for chemically induced seizures (Jobe et al., 1999). Second reason is that the manifestations of forced normalization emerge in epileptic patients as an increasing occurrence of depressive symptoms when the frequency of seizures decreases.

Next to a response to anticonvulsant therapy worsening of affective disorders or psychotic episodes due to the sharply reduced number of seizures postsurgically also may occur (Jobe et al. 1999; Kanner and Balabanov, 2002). Some investigators now believe that antidepressant therapy is crucial for significant number of patients after surgical treatment of epilepsy and that the symptoms of interictal dysphoric disorder tend to occur as chronic seizure activity is suppressed (Jobe et al. 1999; Kanner and Balabanov, 2002).

There is growing body of evidence that anticonvulsant medications have emerged as powerfull agents for the treatment of bipolar disorders, schizoaffective disorder or for the treatment of refractory depression (Jobe et al. 1999; Chaplin et al. 1990; Trimble 1996). On the other side there is an extensive body of evidence that clinically useful antidepressant drugs can both prevent and cause seizures (Jobe et al. 1999; Chaplin et al., 1990; Trimble, 1996). According to contemporary literature antidepressant drugs suppress seizures when blood and brain concentration are relatively low. In contrast to that seizures may occur as a response to antidepressants in overdoses or in response to excessive blood levels (Jobe et al. 1999). Also people with epilepsy exhibit anticonvulsant effects in response to antidepressants and the use of these drugs often represents a safe therapeutic approach in epileptic patients with interictal dysphoric disorder (Jobe et al. 1999).

On the other hand as mentioned above there is a great subgroup of depressive patients and schizophrenic patients without epilepsy which manifest temporal lobe lability and have complex partial seizure-like symptoms with good response to anticonvulsive medication (Roberts et al. 1992; Roberts, 1993; Hines et al. 1995; Bob et al.2005, 2006).

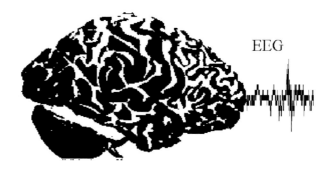

Figure 8. Epileptic or epileptiform EEG activity is characterized by spikes.

2.12. ALTERNATIVE PSYCHOSIS AND DISSOCIATION

Further connection between forced normalization and dissociation represents the term alternative psychosis. From the clinical point of view, forced normalization is often connected with decreasing epileptic changes in EEG and improving the control of seizures. On the other hand for example psychotic symptoms appear. The clinical manifestations of forced normalization also include dysphoric states, hysteria and hypochondria, affective disorders, and miscellanea (twilight states). Forced normalization can be observed in both generalized and partial epilepsies as a rare complication. It is relatively frequently observed in adults with persistent absence seizures (Wolf, 1991; Kanner, 2000, 2001; Schmitz et al.,1999; Marsh and Rao, 2002). Because the term forced normalization is often considered in connection with EEG, Tellenbach in 1965 introduced in this connection the term alternative psychosis implicating that stopping seizures does not mean vanishing or inactivity of the pathological state (Wolf and Trimble, 1985; Krishnamoorthy et al., 2002). Several studies suggest that in the patients who display alternative psychosis subcortical epileptic discharges are continuously present (Wolf and Trimble, 1985). Heath (1962, 1975) pointed out that at the level of subcortical structures epilepsy and manifestations of psychotic symptoms in certain cases might have the same neurobiological substrate in the form of epileptic activity.

Similar findings reported also other authors (Monroe, 1982; Walter, 1944; Goon et al. 1973; Alvarez, 2001), who reported that manifestations of schizophrenic pathology are correlated by subcortical spikes. Reported cases of epileptic seizure, as a consequence of electroconvulsive therapy or other convulsive methods that leads to improvement of psychotic symptoms, points to effects of forced normalization also in cases of "pure" psychosis or depression and it suggest common neurobiological mechanisms between mental illness and epilepsy. Similarly, epileptic discharges located in subcortical structures were observed also in patients with dissociative seizures (Wieser, 1979) which strongly suggest that clear boundary cannot be determined between dissociative and epileptic seizures and that common pathophysiological process for dissociation and epilepsy might be found. At this time the pathogenesis of forced normalization is still unresolved. It has been postulated that amygdaloid and limbic kindling may play a role in the development of this phenomenon and also several neurochemical changes that accompany forced normalization were found (Krishnamoorthy et al. 2002). A more comprehensive hypothesis is that the epilepsy is still active subcortically and provides energy for psychopathological symptoms (Wolf, 1991), and it has often been postulated that subcortical and subclinical electrophysiological activity, particularly in the limbic system, may be responsible for the development of forced normalization (Krishnamoorthy et al. 2002). It is likely that secondary epileptogenesis and other related phenomena may enable continuing of epileptiform activity in limbic areas with predominant psychopathological manifestations (Smith and Darlington, 1996; Stevens, 1992, 1999; Krishnamoorthy et al. 2002).

These alterations and co-occurrence of symptoms are similar to certain conditions that occur during dissociative states when traumatic stress may emerge in a variety of symptoms such as psychopathological symptoms, seizures or other somatoform disturbances. Because dissociation is at least in several reported cases linked to epileptic activity common neurobiological mechanisms of traumatic stress and epileptic activity likely could be present. Modern formulation of dissociation in the terms of discrete behavioral states seems to be able to link cognitive processes related to dissociation and multi-stable perception of ambiguous stimuli with neural network model of dissociative states. Agreement of these conceptual approaches enables to reformulate the concept of dissociation in neuroscientific terms that may include also organic etiology of these pathological conditions.

Frequent occurrence of epileptic activity and epileptiform abnormalities in dissociative states and disorders suggests that close relationship between epileptic activity and kindling might have crucial importance for understanding of dissociative processes. Kindling mechanism caused by stress may involve typical inhibitory failure related to caused by overloading of defensive mechanisms such as denial or "repression" that has been conceptualized for understanding dissociative states (Yates and Nasby, 1993). This process therefore leads to similar lack of inhibiton as epilepsy and therefore it may also cause similar pathological electrophysiological changes as found in epilepsy. Preliminary findings suggest that mental stress may cause increased chaos and neural complexity (Redington and Reidbord, 1992, Bob, 2007), and thqt repeated stress leading to neural chaos may hypothetically represent neurophysiological mechanism inducing epileptic activity as a typical form of chaotic process (Bob et al. 2006). This implicates that dissociation is not synonymous as epileptic activity but in agreement with these findings we may consider the hypothesis that reported relationship between dissociation and epileptic activity might represent manifestation of underlying mechanims related to neural chaos.

2.13. TRAUMATIC STRESS, KINDLING AND TEMPORO-LIMBIC ASYMMETRY

Reported evidence that confirms the relationship of temporal lobe abnormalities and pathological dissociation (Ahern et al., 1993; Putnam, 1997; Sierra and Berrios, 1998; Teicher et al., 2003; Bob, 2003b) in non-epileptic conditions is consistent with data that the dissociative symptoms in temporal lobe epileptics occur during interictal periods and not during the ictal state (Spiegel, 1991). The relationship between dissociation and epileptic activity likely may explain influence of repeated stressful events that lead to an increase in responsivencss to a stress stimuli resulting from repeated stressors with kindling-like progression (Post et al., 1995; Putnam, 1997; Teicher et al., 2003). The kindling-model of stress-related sensitization also seems to be in agreement with suggestive evidence that stress may influence significantly increased occurrence of EEG abnormalities (Teicher et al., 2003; 2006).

There are good reasons for using limbic kindling as a model of epileptogenesis in focal human limbic epilepsy or complex partial seizures with secondary generalization (Adamec, 1990, 1997; Albright and Burnham, 1980; Loscher et al., 1986). This concept is supported by findings of repeated electrical stimulation in human hippocampus and thalamus that caused an epileptic disorder, which was not present before the experiment (Adamec, 1990, 1997; Sramka et al., 1977; Monroe, 1982). Another reason is the evidence that time-dependent spread of epileptic excitability occurs independently on tissue pathology as a consequence of organic damages (Adamec, 1990, 1997; Jensen and Baram, 2000). According to some findings damage creates kindling stimulus that leads to a seizure disorder and the delay between trauma and onset of seizures in humans is consistent with the hypothesis (Adamec, 1990). These findings are also supported by reported cases of successful prophylactic anticonvulsant therapy following head trauma with neurological signs of brain damage that reduce the incidence of an epileptic disorder development (Adamec, 1990, 1997; Servit and Musil, 1981).

Kindling may be also used as a concept for explanation of psychopathological processes as a mirror of altered limbic functions. In manic depressive psychosis the role of kindling was hypothesized in the study of influence of carbamazepin on mood and its anticonvulsant and antikindling effect, which is in agreement with the anticonvulsant effect of carbamazepin in complex partial seizures (Adamec, 1990, 1997). Likely the effectiveness of carbamazepin in the treatment of manic depressive disorder in nonepileptics is due to its limbic anticonvulsant properties that suggest limbic neural mechanism underlying manic depressive disorder (Adamec, 1990, 1997; Dalby, 1975). Dopaminergic hypothesis of schizophrenia provides similar results that show schizophrenic symptoms as consequences of hyperdopaminergic kindling in mesolimbic dopaminergic system (Adamec, 1990, 1997). Some findings also suggest the effect of limbic seizures on dopaminergic functions (Adamec, 1990, 1997) and a relationship of reciprocity between that kindling in mesolimbic dopaminergic and similar EEG activity in temporal neocortex in patients with temporal lobe epilepsy (Pakalnis et al., 1988).

The concept of kindling as a model for psychopathology is also in accordance with recent findings that schizophrenia as well as depression are related to a loss of physiological balance between excitation and inhibition (Stevens, 1999). The significant loss of physiological equilibrium is observed also in epilepsy that is linked to over-excitation whereas schizophrenia as well as depression are likely connected to over-inhibition in the structures of the limbic system. In epilepsy, the normal equilibrium between excitation and inhibition permanently alters by repeated focal excitation or kindling, resulting in a permanent state of excessive focal excitability and spontaneous seizures (Stevens 1999; Goddard et al., 1969). Recent findings indicate that similar "kindling" or sensitization may originate in inhibitory systems in response to focal physiological pulsed discharges of limbic and hypothalamic neurons and this excess of inhibitory factors may then manifest as a psychosis (Stevens, 1992, 1999). Similar situation is also in depression because of decreased activity of serotonin, norepinephrine, dopamine, and GABA that may facilitate the kindling process (Kanner and Balabanov, 2002).

These findings are in accordance with reported cases of forced normalization or alternative psychosis in which decreasing epileptic symptomatology is linked to increased psychopathology in the form of psychosis or depression and vice versa (Jobe et al., 1999; Krishnamoortthy et al., 2002). The kindling in inhibitory systems might also explain occurrence of complex partial seizure-like symptoms in psychiatric patients because of close relationship among traumatic stress, dissociation and complex partial seizure-like symptoms (Bob et al., 2007; Bob et al., 2005, 2006a). These data suggest the relevance of the kindling model of dissociative states as a consequence of repeated traumatic stress (Post et al., 1995; Putnam, 1997) in various psychiatric conditions such as depression or schizophrenia.

Above findings support the kindling hypothesis for explanation of several neurobiological mechanisms of repeated traumatic stress in etiopathogenesis of psychiatric disorders and are also in accordance with published data that document lateralized temporal-limbic dysfunction in patients with schizophrenia and depression, likely caused by subclinical electrophysiological dysfunction (Hugdahl, 2001). According to findings by Gruzelier and Venables different schizophrenic syndromes may be related to asymmetry of limbic functioning and overactivation most probably in the left hemisphere (Gruzelier and Venables, 1974; Gruzelier, 1983). Flor-Henry (1969) reported asymmetries of bilateral electrodermal activity (EDA) in schizophrenia in the form of observable differences between the left- and right-hand recordings and described an association between dysfunction in the left temporal lobe and schizophrenia which has been supported also by recent brain imaging studies (Hugdahl, 2001). Flor-Henry also found that psychotic patients with predominantly schizophrenic symptoms had a high incidence of epileptic foci in the left temporal lobe while depressive patients had a high incidence of foci in the right temporal lobe (Flor-Henry, 2003; Hugdahl, 2001). This association between unilateral hemispheric dysfunction, ipsilateral temporal-limbic epileptic focus (Flor-Henry, 2003; Shulman, 2003; Hugdahl, 2001) and EDA asymmetry is in accordance with recent evidence that EDA is governed mainly by limbic modulation influences and correlates with amygdala activity (Mangina and Beuzeron-Mangina, 1996; Critchley, 2002; Phelps et al., 2001). Additionally, recent data reported in intracranial study by Mangina and Beuzeron-Mangina (1996) indicate that increased activity in the limbic structures caused by electrical stimulation relates to increased ipsilateral EDA.

EDA asymmetry in the patients with temporal epilepsy is in agreement with findings of unilateral electrophysiological dysfunction that predominantly occurs on the left (dominant hemisphere) in schizophrenia and on the right (non-dominant) in depression (Dawson et al., 2000; Hugdahl, 2001). With respect to similar findings in epileptic patients with left or right temporal foci related to schizophrenia and depression, reported EDA dysfunction, predominantly on the left in schizophrenia and on the right in depression, may relate to epileptic-like activity and kindling (Flor-Henry, 1969, 2003). Because of the great sensitivity of EDA on emotional stress, it is possible to suppose that traumatic stress in schizophrenia and depression is related to electrodermal dysfunction because of the asymmetry that was not observed in the healthy control group (Bob et al., 2007c,d,e). These findings support possible relationship between temporal-limbic dysfunction measured by EDA and traumatic stress related to sensitization and kindling mechanism. Results of these studies are also in accordance with recent findings that schizophrenia and depression have a close relationship to a loss of physiological balance between excitation and inhibition, which leads to autonomic hyperarousal in paranoid schizophrenia and hypoarousal in depression.

The findings discussed above in the context of kindling, traumatic stress and dissociation might explain lateralized right hemispheric sympathetic under-activation in depression or left hemispheric sympathetic over-activation in schizophrenia because of asymmetric autonomic control within the brain. The left hemisphere affects predominantly parasympathetic functions, while the right hemisphere predominantly governs the sympathetic functions (Hilz et al., 2001; Avnon et al., 2004). This is in accordance with several findings in schizophrenia, which suggest that psychotic states affect the autonomic nervous system and suppress the parasympathetic function without affecting sympathetic function (Toichi et al., 1999; Takahashi et al., 2005). These data are consistent with the above hypothesis of the kindling in inhibitory systems because of repeated emotional disturbances. Lateralized activation of left-sided inhibition in schizophrenia due to kindling may lead to suppression of parasympathetic function without affecting sympathetic function and vice versa in depression in which right-sided inhibition may lead to suppression of sympathetic function without affecting parasympathetic function as is evident from electrodermal measures indicating lowering of sympathetic activity in depression. This interpretation is consistent with several findings that emotional stress may lead to two predominant forms of stress response. The first form of stress response leads to predominant sympathetic influences and the second form of stress response relates to predominant parasympathetic functions (Ul'yaninskii, 1995; Mason et al., 2001). This corresponds to known experience that mainly chronic stress often leads to a passive defense and predominant parasympathetic influences on neuroendocrine metabolic activity.

2.14. DISSOCIATION AND HEMISPHERIC LATERALITY

Important concept in the history of understanding dissociation is also Cerebral Hemispheric Laterality Model. The model represents the theory that either an anatomical or a functional disconnection between the two hemispheres of the brain is the source of "double personality" (Putnam, 1989, 1997; Ellenberger, 1970; Quen, 1986). Competitive inter-hemispheric alter personality states connected to dissociated mental representations of corresponding neural assemblies thus suggest the explanation of repeated clinical observations that document laterality differences across alter personalities in multiple personality patients (Brende, 1982, 1984; Henninger, 1992; Le Page et al., 1992; Ahern, 1993; Putnam, 1984, 1997). For example, Ahern et al. (1993) examined the relationship of "multiple personality disorder" in two patients with temporolimbic epilepsy to certain types of hemispheric interaction. Both patients exhibited different "personalities" in a characteristic temporal relationship to their seizures. These two patients with temporolimbic epilepsy were considered to be surgical candidates referred for the intracarotid amobarbital sodium procedure. Both patients have demonstrated outbursts of emotional behaviour during inactivation of the left hemisphere. These "different personalities" were known to the patient's families to manifest themselves in the postictal period. These observations suggest that the association of multiple personality and temporolimbic epilepsy is not dependent on seizure discharges per se, but rather may be related to certain types of hemispheric interaction (Ahern et al., 1993).

On the other hand there are controlled test of the laterality that did not find evidence of shifts in lateralization of galvanic skin response across repeatedly randomized testing of alter-personality states (Putnam, 1997) that are not bound to inter-hemispheric competition.

This suggests that competition between dissociated alter personalities and their neural representations may course in the form of intra-hemispheric as well as inter-hemispheric competition. This depends on the predominant qualities of competitive alter personalities. For example, when the first alter will have left hemispheric dominance and the second right hemispheric dominance then the identity shift will be linked to laterality differences. When both alter personalities will have right (respectively left) hemispheric dominance then the identity shift will not be connected to laterality differences.

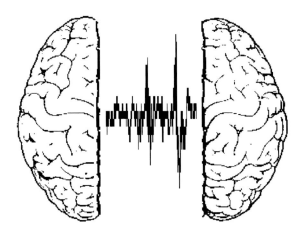

Figure 9. Interaction of dissociated hemispheres could be functionally linked to epileptiform activity.

2.15. TRAUMATIC STRESS AND INTER-HEMISPHERIC DYSFUNCTION

Above reviewed findings on hemispheric laterality in dissociative states suggest that traumatic stress may influence patterns of brain asymmetry and interhemispheric dysregulation. It is in agreement with recent findings that the right hemisphere is more vulnerable to traumatic influences than the left (Henry, 1993, 1997). Reason for that is likely increased right hemispheric connection with the limbic system in comparison with the left hemisphere. The right (more often non-dominant) hemisphere is also more connected with autonomic nervous system and has predominant role in the physiological and cognitive aspects of emotional processing and is more than the left specialized for neuroendocrine and autonomic activation, for the secretion of the stress hormones, corticotrophin releasing factors and cortisol (Spence et al., 1996; Sullivan and Gratton, 1999a,b; Wittling and Pfluger,

1990; Schore, 2001, 2002). Evidence for this lateralization provide studies dealing with the relationship between conditioned fear response and amygdala function, which show that this activation is right hemisphere dominant (LaBar et al., 1998). Also has been reported that partial kindling of the right and not the left amygdala induces a long-lasting increase in anxiety-like behavior (Adamec, 1997, 1999), and that the kindling in the right amygdala induces increased production of the corticotrophin releasing factors (Adamec and McKay, 1993). Recent evidence also suggests that the right amygdala is more involved in the storage of fearful faces and in the expression of emotionally influenced memory of aversive experiences with respect to the left (Morris et al., 1999; Isenberg et al., 1999; Coleman-Mensches and McGaugh, 1995; Schore, 2002). Certain neuropsychological studies of alexithymia also suggest a right-hemispheric dysfunction linked to a defect of information transfer across the corpus callosum that leads to a physiological disconnection of the two hemispheres and resulting inability to coordinate the affective expression of the right hemisphere with the verbal expression of the left hemisphere (Dewaraja and Sasaki, 1990; Schore, 2001). This dysfunction typically leads to difficulty in verbal expression of emotions "no words for feelings" that is typical for alexithymia. Alexithymia is closely related to dissociation (Kooiman et al., 2004; Sayar et al., 2005; Frewen et al., 2006) and similar defects of information transfer across the corpus callosum in alexithymia (Tabibnia and Zaidel, 2005; Romei et al., 2008) and dissociation has been observed (Spitzer et al., 2004). This hemispheric dysfunction might indicate a relationship between traumatic dissociation on the psychological level and related "functional dissociation" of the hemispheres. This functional dissociation according to literature may be a form of reversible blocking of information transfer across corpus callosum (Bogen and Bogen, 1969). This might explain why certain dissociative symptoms are similar to symptoms in the patients with split brain as a consequence of anatomical "dissociation" between hemispheres which occur after surgical cut of corpus callosum (Ahern et al., 1993; Galin, 1974; Brende, 1984; Bob, 2003b; Bogen and Bogen, 1969; Spitzer et al., 2004). The functional dissociation might be a defense mechanism that enables to health hemisphere to inhibit the negative impulses from the dysfunctional hemisphere, similarly as in psychological dissociation that inhibits a certain negative psychological impulses, which does not fit into current cognitive scheme. In this context Nasrallah (1985) suggested that one of the vital components of interhemispheric integration is the inhibition of any awareness by the verbally expressive hemispheric consciousness (predominantly the left) that it actually receives and sends thoughts, intentions, and feelings from and to another (right hemispheric) consciousness. This inhibition guarantees the unity of the right and left hemispheres into one "self" in the normal person and is disturbed in schizophrenia, because of defective interhemispheric integration that may lead to disinhibition of the awareness by the left hemisphere that it is being "influenced" by an unknown "external force", which is in fact the right hemisphere. Schneiderian delusions such as thought insertion and withdrawal and passivity feelings may be a direct outcome of such a deficit (Nasrallah, 1985). In this context, also Miller (1992) suggested that borderline splitting and borderline pathology may have a neural basis because of split between emotional and cognitive constitution and its lateralization in the brain. Because interhemispheric communication is necessary for mental unity, childhood emotional trauma may cause the two separate, unintegrated and alternating mental systems that are related to congenital abnormality in brain structure or function and may be a primary factor in borderline pathology (Miller, 1992).

Together recent data show that dysregulation in the brain asymmetry and mental functioning may be caused by stress-related activation that can also influence the peripheral endocrine glands through the pituitary gland and also via direct neural pathways between the CNS structures and the target endocrine glands. Recent data suggest that adequate control of the target neuroendocrine structures requires asymmetry of neural regulation and that the patterns of cerebral asymmetry can be retroactively modified by the endocrine glands (Gerendai and Halasz, 2001). Recent data from animal models indicate that there is a functional asymmetry in the medial prefrontal cortex concerning neuroendocrine and autonomic stress responses and that both prestress and acute restraint stress-induced plasma corticosterone levels are lower in animals with right or bilateral lesion of the medial prefrontal cortex (Gerendai and Halasz, 2001; Edwards et al., 2000). In the context of kindling and lateralized epileptiform discharges there are also clinical data suggesting the asymmetry of the temporal lobe in the control of peripheral glands related to reproductive functions. For example, among women with partial seizures of temporal lobe origin, reproductive disorders are unusually common and was found that polycystic ovarian syndrome is predominantly associated with left-sided epileptiform discharges, whereas hypothalamic amenorrhea is related predominantly to right-sided discharges (Herzog, 1993; Gerendai and Halasz, 2001). These data suggest that also relationship between stress and kindling may potentially explain various dysfunctions and diseases related to disturbed asymmetry in neuroendocrine regulation.

An important aspect of the present findings is lateralized regulation of stress responses at the level of the mPFC that indicates close relationship between stress or emotionality-related processes and right brain mechanisms (Sullivan and Gratton, 1999a,b, 2002). Prelimbic and infralimbic regions of mPFC have an influence to visceral motor regions, autonomic functions and emotional expression, and present an important region for the integration of neuroendocrine and autonomic activity with the behavioral states and cognitive processes (Sullivan and Gratton, 1999a,b, 2002). These studies suggest that although the right mPFC is necessary for a normal stress response and adaptation, excessive activity of this region is predominantly maladaptive. Further research regarding relationship between stress exposure and the level of neuropsychological, autonomic and neuroendocrine asymmetry may perspectively show other possible connections of these processes to excessive epileptic-like neural activity that may present common neural mechanism of various levels of the stress response because of increased neural excitability and dysregulated asymmetry in neural activity patterns.

Chapter 3

DISSOCIATION AND SCHIZOPHRENIA

3.1. DEMENTIA PRAECOX OR MULTIPLE PERSONALITY DISORDER?

In 1911 Eugen Bleuler in his work *Dementia praecox or the group of the schizophrenias*, introduced the new term to describe this serious illness that replaced Kraepelin's term dementia praecox. In his Text-book of psychiatry he wrote (Bleuler, 1924): "It is not alone in hysteria that one finds an arrangement of different personalities one succeeding the other. Through similar mechanism schizophrenia produces different personalities existing side by side." (p. 138). The process of splitting in schizophrenia is according to Bleuler (Bleuler 1924; Rosenbaum, 1980; Bottero, 2001; Scharfetter, 1998) the same as splitting of psychic connections in hysteria and in an extreme version it can lead to the emergence of alter personalities and typical amnesia. These important Bleuler's ideas regarding the notion of schizophrenia are historically related to the concept of dissociation developed by Pierre Janet (Janet, 1890; Ellenberger, 1970; van der Hart and Friedman, 1989; Bob, 2003a, Read et al. 2001; Ross 2004). Etiology of schizophrenia is thus traditionally explained by Bleuler along the lines of Pierre Janet as being a consequence of dissociative reaction (Ellenberger 1970), analogous to somnambulism, fugue states, hypnosis or psychogenic amnesia. Dissociative reaction is most often a consequence of abuse or traumatic experiences leading to a loss of the inhibitory control of certain mental contents that may lead to the production of split fragments of the psyche due to abnormal intensive negative affect. Pierre Janet, in his work about psychological automatisms (Janet, 1890; Ellenberger, 1970; van der Hart and Friedman, 1989), defines dissociation as being a defect of the associated system that creates the secondary consciousness, which he called the subconscious fixed idea. Similarly, Sigmund Freud and Joseph Breuer considered secondary consciousness in "Studies in hysteria" (Breuer and Freud, 1895). Because Janet used the term dissociation to denote a splitting of the psyche and on the contrary Bleuler and Jung used the term dissociation as a synonym for splitting, historical roots for the same meaning of splitting and dissociation are evident (Bleuler, 1911/1955; Jung, 1909; Ellenberger, 1970). Similar relationship is also between structural descriptions of the subconscious fixed idea defined by Janet and the psychic complex comprehensively described by Jung (Ellenberger, 1970; Jung, 1909). Jung in his research on complexes confirmed Janet's findings of the dissociability of consciousness and the potentiality of a personality disintegration into fragments (Jung, 1972a). Similarly Bleuler in his "Consciousness and Associations" described complexes analogically to Janet's description of fixed ideas and wrote that there is "no difference in principle between unconscious complexes and these several personalities endowed with consciousness" because of increasing number of disturbed associations with the ego as a whole (Bleuler, 1918/1906, p. 291). Similarly in the recent literature the fixed idea is described as a formation of new spheres of consciousness around memories of intensely arousing experiences with a high emotional charge, which organize cognitive, affective and visceral elements of the traumatic experience while simultaneously keeping them out of conscious awareness (van der Hart and Friedman, 1989). It is analogical to the definition of the complex as an organized collection of ideas, emotions, impulses and memories that share a common emotional tone, and have been excluded partly or entirely from consciousness but continue to influence a person's thoughts, emotions and behavior (Colman, 2003).

The term complex was introduced by Theodor Ziehen, who used this term in the late 1890s for explanation of prolonged reaction time in the word association test as a reaction to something unpleasant for the subject (Ellenberger, 1970). Jung elaborated the theory of psychic complexes in his experiments in Burghölzl and described them in his studies of word associations (Jung 1968, 1972b,c, 1973). When a defect occurs in free associations it is caused by a complex (Jung 1907, 1968, 1972b,c, 1973). According to Jung's findings the complex always has its own autonomy and behaves as a split part of the psyche. When a complex is evoked into the consciousness, its physiological or pathological influence depends on a degree of its autonomy or, contrary to that, compatibility with other complexes respective to the ego-complex. In the case of pathological influence the complex leads to a lowered mental level, (*abaissement du niveau mental*) (Janet, 1890; Ellenberger, 1970; van der Hart and Friedman, 1989; Bob, 2003a).

The fundamental causes of the etiology of pathological dissociated fixed ideas or complexes, as Janet suggested, are mainly traumatic events, which produce traumatic memories. Complexes thus generate alternate fields of the psyche, and it is possible, by means of these complexes, to explain also extreme cases which occur in multiple personality disorder (Bob, 2004). In the *The Psychology of the Dementia Praecox*, Jung experimentally demonstrated a dynamic concept of schizophrenia based on the theory of dissociated complexes (Jung, 1909; Ellenberger, 1970). He applied the associative experiment to schizophrenic subjects and compared these results to experiments performed in normal persons. These experiments led him to define a condition of inner distraction determined by a complex. The condition is analogical to Weygandt's term "apperceptive deterioration" and is closely related to the concept of "abaissement du niveau mental" proposed by Janet as the cause of dissociation (Jung, 1909; Ellenberger, 1970; Bob, 2003a; Shin et al., 2005; Bovensiepen 2006). Jung's experimental findings in neurotic and psychotic patients as well as in normal persons have documented material supporting Bleuler's clinical hypothesis regarding the common mechanisms underlying the formation of symptoms in hysteria and the symptoms of dementia praecox (Jung, 1909; Ellenberger, 1970; Bob et al., 2006). According to Jung, during schizophrenia the psyche is split-off into a plurality of autonomous complexes and the whole personality is pathologically disintegrated.

Later after the Second World War this conceptual overlap was neglected mainly because of formation of biological theories of schizophrenia that caused distraction from psychological understanding of schizophrenia. Nevertheless this conceptual overlap still survived in clinical diagnostics as suggest a review of Index Medicus from 1903 to the revival of interest in multiple personality in 1978 that shows a dramatic decline in the number of reports of multiple personality, which indicates that many patients with multiple personality had been diagnosed and treated as schizophrenics (Rosenbaum, 1980; Foote and Park, 2008). It is in agreement with findings that a substantial number of patients with dissociative identity disorder have previous diagnoses of schizophrenia (Rosenbaum, 1980; Elason and Ross, 1995). It is mainly due to a presence of positive symptoms of schizophrenia in patients with multiple personality disorder (or dissociative identity disorder in DSM IV) that report more positive symptoms of schizophrenia than schizophrenics. It is important to note that schizophrenics report more negative symptoms and therefore a primary emphasis on positive symptoms may result in false-positive diagnoses of schizophrenia and false-negative diagnoses of dissociative identity disorder (Elason and Ross, 1995). On the other hand there are findings that show markedly high level of dissociation in schizophrenic patients (Bernstein and Putnam, 1986; Read et al. 2001; Spitzer et al. 1997; Startup, 1999; Merckelbach et al., 2000; Morrison et al., 2003; Glaslova et al., 2004; Bob et al., 2006a). These data are also in agreement with findings that suggest significant influence of stress in etiopathogenesis of schizophrenia (Walker and Diforio, 1997; Boksa and El-Khodor, 2003; Corcoran et al., 2003).

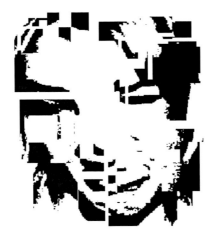

Figure 10. Dissociated mind in schizophrenia.

3.2. BINDING PROBLEM AND SCHIZOPHRENIA

Modern findings suggest that disturbances of integrity or dissociative processes in schizophrenia occur due to similar disturbances of integrity at the level of brain functions mediated by binding of distributed information within the brain (Tononi and Edelman, 2000). Recent increasing experimental evidence suggests that coherent neuronal assemblies in the brain are functionally linked by synchronization between simultaneously recorded EEG signals and that this time-dependent synchrony represents neural substrate for mental representations such as perception, cognitive functions and memory (Braitenberg, 1978; Singer, 1993, 2001; Lachaux et al., 1999; Varela et al., 2001; Fries, 2005). A deficit in the integration of distributed macroscopic patterns of neuronal activity into a coherent whole may be a functional counterpart of defective patterns of interactions among specialized brain areas in schizophrenia (Tononi and Edelman, 2000; Peled, 1999; Lee et al., 2003).

This conscious disintegration probably produces defective self-monitoring and self-experiencing, for example during hallucinations (Feinberg, 1978; Ford et al., 2001, 2007; Poulet and Hedwig, 2007). Using the PET scan was found that applying the same task to people with schizophrenia, and comparing hallucinators to nonhallucinators, show that the hallucinators have decreased flow in the areas used to monitor speech, such as the left middle temporal gyrus and supplementary motor area (Andreasen, 1997).

Recent findings suggest that the disintegration could be caused by defective communication between the frontal lobes, where speech is generated, and the temporal lobes, where it is perceived (Ford et al., 2005). This process likely may occur through the action of corollary discharges (or an efference copy) mechanism that prepares the temporal lobes for the expected sound (Ford et al., 2005).

Already Hughlings Jackson pointed out that also thinking may be considered the highest and most complex motor activity (Feinberg, 1978). This Jackson's clinical finding is in agreement with evidence of defective self-monitoring and self-integrity that originates in research of motor brain structures and from studies of corollary discharges (Feinberg and Guazzelli, 1999).

Motor commands from these brain structures are associated with neural discharges that alter activity in both sensory and motor pathways. These neural discharges called corollary discharges (or efference copy) enables monitoring and modification of the commands themselves before the effector event. They enable to inform sensory systems that the stimulation produced by movement is self-generated or produced by an environment, which is crucial for the distinction of self and non-self (Feinberg, 1978; Ford et al., 2001, 2007; Poulet and Hedwig, 2007). There is evidence that derangement of corollary discharges included in motor mechanisms of thinking produce many symptoms of schizophrenia in the visual or auditory system. Self-generated eye movements generate a "corollary discharge," or "efference copy" of the motor plan, informing the visual cortex that the changing of a visual input results from a self-generated action. A similar mechanism may exist in the auditory system, where corollary discharges from motor speech commands prepare the auditory cortex for self-generated speech, perhaps through a link between frontal lobes, where speech is generated, and temporal lobes, where it is heard (Ford et al., 2001, 2007; Poulet and Hedwig, 2007). These findings provide direct neurophysiological evidence for a corollary discharge that transforms sensory responses to self-generated and relative to externally presented percepts. These percepts fail in patients with schizophrenia in comparison to healthy subjects. For example, inner speech is misidentified as external voices (Ford et al., 2001, 2007; Poulet and Hedwig, 2007).

Loss of distinctions between internally generated psychic activity and external input is crucial for dissociative states as were formulated by Janet and also for the dreamy states defined by Hughlings Jackson (Meares, 1999). Dissociation represents disturbances of self-identity when own psychic contents are splitted and disintegrated from consciousness by dissociative mechanism, and create the co-conscious (or unconscious) level of psychic functioning (Bob, 2007b).

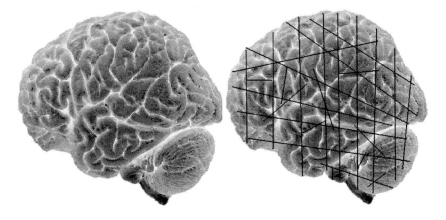

Figure 11. Brain integrity and dissociation.

Chapter 4

DISSOCIATION AND "WOUNDED MIND"

4.1. DISSOCIATION AND TRAUMATIC STRESS

Dissociation represents a special form of consciousness in which events that would ordinarily be connected are divided from one another (Li and Spiegel, 1992) or it is also often less generally understood as inability to integrate some psychic contents into the consciousness (Bernstein and Putnam, 1986). Dissociation is defined in DSM-III-R and DSM-IV as "a disturbance or alteration in the normally integrative functions of identity, memory or consciousness" and leads also to characteristic somatoform changes (Nijenhuis et al. 1996) such as alterations in sensation of pain (analgesia, kinesthetic anesthesia), painful symptoms, perception alterations, motor inhibition or loss of motor control, gastrointestinal symptoms and dissociative seizures (Brown and Trimble 2000; Kuyk et al. 1999).

The group of syndromes which are immediately bound to dissociative processes were elaborated by John Nemiah (1981). Main features are these: 1. alteration of identity as a consequence of dissociative reaction and 2. disturbance of memory of an individual during dissociative states. These principles were used for the first definition of diagnostic classification of dissociative states in the DSM III frame. The third important principle defined by Putnam (1989) is based on experiences from the study of dissociative reaction where the major part of dissociative disorders was induced by traumatic events. The most important traumas originate in childhood due to physical or sexual abuse with following development of symptoms often after many years. Dissociative symptoms also frequently occur due to traumatic event after serious accidents or natural calamities. Symptoms of disintegration often develop in the connection to posttraumatic stress disorder (Spiegel and Cardena, 1991). Characteristic features of these dissociative symptoms are changes in notion of identity as depersonalization or in serious cases multiple personality disorder. Another experienced symptoms represent changes in notion of external world such as derealization, hallucinations or changes of memory, for example psychogenic amnesia or multiple personality disorder (Spiegel and Cardena, 1991). For example Chu and Dill (1990) investigated dissociation by means of Dissociative Experiences Scale (DES) in 98 females and found significantly higher dissociation in patients who were exposed to emotional or physical abuse. Coons, Bowman and Pellow (1989), in their study of prevalence of traumas in childhood and adult clinical population, found that 100% patients with atypical dissociative disorders and 82% diagnosed as psychogenic amnesia documented physical or verbal abuse or neglect in childhood. About half of patients experienced also significant trauma in adulthood. Briere and Conte (1989) have documented that 59,6% from the group of 468 patients with proven history of sexual abuse in childhood were not able to remember the episodes of abuse from the past. There is growing evidence that child abuse is a very important factor in many psychiatric disorders and that dissociative symptomatology often occurs due to child abuse especially in cases of chronic emotional, physical or sexual abuse (Spiegel and Cardena, 1991; Putnam, 1997, Teicher et al. 2003; Sar and Ross, 2006).

Together these findings suggest that any exposed or reported trauma may be important for the development of dissociative symptomatology and may be closely related to many symptoms such as depresssion, hallucinations and other. On the other hand it is necessary to mention that in ICD-10 is also defined the organic dissociation that relates to dissociative symptoms and disorders including amnesia, fugue, depersonalization, multiple personality, automatisms, and certain furors which can be induced by a variety of medications, abuse of drugs, and medical illnesses or conditions affecting cerebral functions. It is important to note that organic dissociation can be distinguished from intoxication, amnestic disorder, and delirium (Good, 1993). Conversely, it is important that dissociation as a reaction to psychological stressors and traumas has various neurobiological consequences (Teicher et al., 2003, 2006; Putnam, 1997). Repeated stressors and reexperiencing of the traumatic event in childhood often cause the delayed effects of severe psychological trauma that lead to enhancement of the self-preservative catecholamine states related to anger, fear, meaninglessness and a blunting of the emotional responses of the attachment behavior associated with dysfunction of the locus coeruleus, amygdala and hippocampal systems (Henry, 1992, 1997). The functional defects in the hippocampus lead to decreasing inhibitory control of the hippocampus on the HPA axis and cause a positive feedforward cascade of glucocorticoide levels (Bao et al., 2008). Recent data indicate that most serious disturbances of HPA axis caused by traumatic events such as childhood abuse or neglect in the first years of life often have long-term impact on emotional, behavioral, cognitive, social and physiological functions and vice versa love and social care also may influence these functions and improve dissociative disturbances (Horowitz et al., 1979; Ito et al., 1998; Heim et al., 2000; Orr and Roth, 2000; Teicher et al. 2003; Read et al., 2001; Esch and Stefano 2007; Stefano and Esch, 2007). These neuroendocrinological and neurophysiological dysfunctions related to trauma cause memory disturbances, dissociation and also a variety of somatic symptoms that have a profound role in the long-term adaptation to traumatic experience and lead to a lack of integration of somatoform components of experience, reactions, and functions (Nijenhuis et al., 1996, 2004; Nijenhuis, 2000; Bowman and Coons, 2000). From ethological point of view there are clinical experiences that dissociation could be a parallel process to animal defensive and recuperative states that are evoked in the face of severe threat. Empirical data and clinical observations seem to be supportive of the idea that there are similarities between freezing, concomitant development of analgesia and anesthesia, and acute pain in threatened animals (Nijenhuis et al., 1998). These primary defense strategies supported by the parasympathetic nervous system involve energy conservation that cause passive coping strategies such as withdrawal or disengagement, dissociation, and the immobility response (Schore, 1994, 2001). Typical emotions associated with parasympathetic functions have a negative valence, such as shame, disgust, hopelessness, and despair (Schore, 1994, 2001). Dissociation is an analogical form of human response to inescapable and threatening stress with the same defensive tendency toward passive and avoidant coping that emerge as hopelessness, learned helplessness, social and emotional withdrawal and disengagement (van der Kolk et al., 1985; Nijenhuis et al., 1998, 2004).

4.2. DISSOCIATION AND MEMORY

Recent findings suggest that dissociation is not only pathological but it also has some adaptive functions and that dissociative phenomena occur in the normal population (Putnam, 1989). On the other hand in most cases of pathological dissociation, the loss of episodic and/or emotional memories is related to traumatic stress, nevertheless brain insult, injury or other organic brain disease may play a role in this process (Kihlstrom, 2005; Spiegel, 1997). Although in ICD-10 is also defined the organic dissociation, induced by a variety of conditions affecting cerebral function (Good, 1993), dissociative disorders are mainly induced due to a traumatic event (Sar and Ross, 2006; Brewin, 2007; Bob, 2008).

Dysfunctions in accessibility of memory traces that represents traumatic and other negative past experiences as well as intrusive autobiographical memories of childhood abuse are closely related to an effort to eliminate these negative memories and increases intrusive thoughts connected to inner conflict due to contradictory tendencies when unacceptable or traumatic memory is released to the consciousness. Disturbed temporal memory related to stress conditions is evident from studies focused on episodic and autobiographical memories. For example, results in the group of eighty-seven children aged 7-15 years exposed to a traumatic event requiring hospitalization indicate that specifically children who showed temporal disorganization, but not absence of emotion or dissociative amnesia, in narrative themes were more likely to report concurrent subsyndromal PTSD symptoms at 4-7 weeks post-trauma (Kenardy et al., 2007). Similarly other results show experiments demonstrating that exposure to a significant psychological stressor preserves or even enhances memory for emotional aspects of an event, and simultaneously disrupts memory for non-emotional aspects of the same event (Payne et al., 2006).

There is also well documented that individuals who are victims of a trauma are unable to register pain (for example during self-injury) or painful affects (Butler, Duran, Jasiukaitis, Koopman and Spiegel, 1996; Frankel, 1996; Agargun, Tekeoglu, Kara, Adak, and Ercan, 1998; Ebrinc, 2002; Trief, 1996; Saxe, Chawla and van der Kolk, 2002; Russr, Shearin, Clarkin, Harrison and Hull, 1993; Orbach, Mikulincer, King, Cohen and Stein, 1997). Patients with dissociative disorders frequently report amnesia for self-injury (Saxe, Chawla and van der Kolk, 2002; Putnam, 1989). This is due to profound changes in affect state, memory and sense of identity in response to environmental stress injury (Saxe, Chawla and van der Kolk, 2002). According to recent evidence memory may be disturbed by biological as well as psychological traumatic insults that may lead to retrograde amnesia– compatible to Ribot's Law– and a variety of brain disorders such as psychogenic amnesia, multiple personality disorder, hysteria and other dissociative phenomena. At this point the findings about dissociation and traumatic memories represent important empirical material which provides substantial data for the investigations based on experimental memory research.

Historical and recent findings indicate that repeated stress and especially traumatic stress experiences may disturb mental integrity and lead to dissociation of memory and mental experience (Bob, 2003a; Putnam, 1997; van der Hart and Friedman, 1989; Spiegel and Cardena, 1991; Spiegel, 1997; Brewin, 2007). This clinical experience of psychological fragmentation of memory contents is in agreement with experimental evidence of the neural dissociability of the memory processes (Phillips and LeDoux 1992, LeDoux 1992, 1993, 1994; Nadel, 1994). The evidence supports the view that memory systems concerned with encoding emotion and context are dissociable at psychological, physiological, and anatomical levels (Bechara et al. 1995).

Recent findings suggest that memory and neural dissociability is closely related to memory consolidation and could be explained in the framework of this process. Memory consolidation is defined as the process by which recent memories contained in short-term memory are transformed into long-term memory (Debiec, Doyere, Nader, and LeDoux, 2006). This process on the molecular level is linked to protein synthesis that requires involvement of transcription factors CREB and brain derived neurotrophic factor (BDNF) and other molecular processes (see below) that enable global process of network consolidation mainly in the hippocampus but also in other structures (Debiec, Doyere, Nader, and LeDoux, 2006; Debiec, LeDoux, and Nader, 2002; Lee, Everitt, and Thomas, 2004). According to recent findings the amygdala also participates in modulation of memory consolidation and likely has a specific role in consolidation of the traumatic memory (Cahill, 1997; Cahill and McGaugh, 1998). Consolidation of the traumatic memory has certain specific psychological and neurophysiological characteristics (Nadel and Jacobs, 1998; Bob, 2007a). The traumatic memory is not acceptable for conscious awareness because of coupled strong negative emotions. Extremely negative emotion experience during the traumatic event may lead to atypical memory consolidation characterized by consolidation process predominantly on implicit (subliminal) level that produce dissociated state of memory that does not fit into conscious cognitive scheme. This consolidation on implicit level may be caused by inescapable stress which may block the induction of long-term potentiation in medial prefrontal cortex (PFC) and hippocampus. This blocking of higher-order behavior mediated by hippocampus and PFC allows more automatic responses dependent on subcortical structures, mainly the amygdala (Maroun and Richter-Levin, 2003). These findings are also in accordance with neuroimaging data which suggest that characteristic changes in the perfusion of limbic brain structures, such as the amygdala and the hippocampus, coincide with the high arousal and/or anxiety during traumatic recall (Vermetten and Bremner, 2004). High anxiety and arousal are thought to extremely focus the attention and this attentional shift may produce fragmented memories, personality fragmentation (Vermetten and Bremner, 2004; Bob, 2007a), psychological automatisms and lowering of mental level as described by Janet (Putnam, 1997; Bob, 2003a). These data also implicate important consequences for psychotherapy that must enable memory reconsolidation in safe and non-dangerous conditions, which lead to neurobiological reprocessing of memory traces. This reconditioning and reconsolidation is therefore possible only by re-experiencing of the traumatic memory in a new and safe situation during psychotherapeutic process which enables integration of the dissociative state (Bob, 2007a), For example, reconsolidation process of the dissociated traumatic memory during hypnosis that enables efficient memory facilitation (Wagstaff et al., 2004) probably serves as neurobiological mechanism of hypnotic abreaction (Bob, 2007a). During this process implicitly consolidated traumatic memory in subcortical structures, mainly in the amygdala, is probably transformed from automatic into higher level of conscious experience by long-term potentiation in the higher-level structures of CNS such as medial PFC and hippocampus. These results are consistent with other findings of differential effects of stress on brain systems responsible for encoding and retrieving emotional memories in the amygdala and non-emotional memories in the hippocampal formation. Together these findings indicate that memories formed under high levels of stress are not qualitatively the same as those formed under ordinary emotional circumstances but display typical forms of disorganization, fragmentation and incompleteness (Payne et al., 2006; Brewin, 2007).

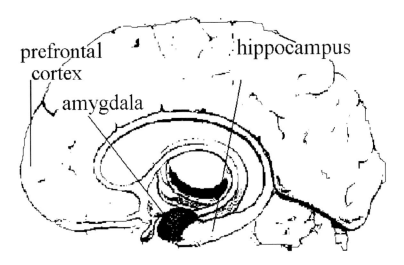

Figure 12. Memory structures of the brain.

Without memory reconsolidation traumatic recall can not be processed in an integrated mode of consciousness and released traumatic memory remains dissociated as a discontinuous experience with amnesic gaps. In the case of abreactive experience, the successive reconsolidation provides a process, during which the revivificated traumatic memory gets re-stabilized in its re-integrated form. Neuroscience research of memory and emotional processes during traumatic recall induced by abreactive process strongly suggests that successful therapeutic work with a dissociative state helps the individual both psychologically and physiologically and that measurable physiology is related to these changes induced by psychotherapeutic process (Bob, 2007a). Neural process of reconsolidation in principle may represent potential existence of a new adaptive level in neurophysiological process, which is actualized for example during successful therapy. Memory reconsolidation probably enables successful transformation from dissociated, automatic and implicitly consolidated traumatic memory mainly in the amygdala, to higher level of conscious experience in the higher-level structures such as medial PFC and hippocampus. This view corresponds to Janet's definition of dissociative state as an automatic process which does not fit into current cognitive scheme and without successful reprocessing (or reconsolidation) remains dissociated also during recall of dissociative state (into awareness of dominant ego-state) because of the specific neural substrate of dissociated memories (Bob, 2007a). Because dissociated memories contain also personality fragments and recall of traumatic memory may lead to personality alterations we can understand and describe them as traumatized ego-states (Frederick, 2005; Watkins and Watkins, 1979-80; Watkins, 1993).

4.3. BINDING PROBLEM, TIME CONSCIOUSNESS AND MELATONIN

More than three centuries ago Rene Descartes described the pineal gland as "the seat of the soul." He thought that ". . . although the soul is joined to the whole body there is a certain part where it exercises its functions more than all the others" (Passions of the Soul, p. 31). Descartes used the clock metaphor as an explanation for basic mechanism of the brain and other physiological functions (Barrera-Mera and Barrera-Calva, 1998; Smith, 1998; Bob and Fedor-Freybergh, 2008). He thought that when we sense only one image with two eyes, only one sound with two ears or only one object by two hands, the sensations from two sources must be fused somewhere. Descartes intuitively postulated that this information is fused and governed by clock mechanism in the pineal gland. He believed that the pineal gland is involved in sensation, imagination, memory and the causation of bodily movements, and described the mind as an extracorporeal entity that is expressed through the pineal gland (Barrera-Mera and Barrera-Calva, 1998; Smith, 1998; Bob and Fedor-Freybergh, 2008). In his thought, Descartes intuitively anticipated the so-called "binding problem" of consciousness that means the neural correlate of consciousness as a part of the nervous system that transforms neural activity in reportable subjective experiences. Major hypothesis is that this neural correlate of consciousness can compare and bind activity patterns only if they arrive simultaneously at the neural correlate of conscious experience (van de Grind, 2002). Consciousness combines the present multimodal sensory information with relevant elements of the past and creates spatio-temporal memory. Information from each modality is continuously distributed into distinct features and locally processed in different relatively specialized brain regions and globally integrated by interactions among these regions. Information is represented by integration through levels of synchronization within neuronal populations and of coherence among multiple brain regions that facilitate large-scale integration, or "binding" (John, 2002; Singer, 2001; Crick and Koch, 2003; Zeman, 2001; Bob and Fedor-Freybergh, 2008). In this process of temporal integration and binding a specific and major role play neurons of suprachiasmatic nuclei. These individual neural oscillators with the temporal patterns of rhythmicity are organized into a coherent activity of biological clock and facilitate temporal synchronization that produces differentially timed waves specifically targeting the pineal gland and other structures, and control neuroendocrine rhythms (Kalsbeek et al., 2006; Indic et al., 2007; Hamada et al., 2004). Melatonin as one of the endocrine output signals of the clock provides circadian information as an endogenous synchronizer able to stabilize and reinforce circadian rhythms and to maintain their mutual phase-relationship. This integrative process occurs at the different levels of the circadian network via gene expression in some brain regions and peripheral structures that enables integration of circadian, hormonal, and metabolic information and creating temporal order of bodily and mental experience (Rutter, 2002; Pevet, 2006; Saper, 2005). This specific temporal order is reflected in associative process that is necessary for cognition, behavior and all processes of memory consolidation that must preserve all the information in the temporal causal order and synchrony or sequentiality of the internal cognitive maps. In this context recent findings suggest that melatonin could be a potential regulator in the processes that contribute to memory formation, long-term potentiation (LTP) and synaptic plasticity in the hippocampus and other brain regions (Baydas et al., 2005; Larson et al., 2006; Chaudhury, Wang, and Colwell, 2005; Ozcan, Yilmaz, and Carpenter, 2006; Gorfine and Zisapel, 2007). Basic mechanism of melatonin action is that it may interact with both excitatory and inhibitory neurotransmiter systems (Larson et al., 2006; Saenz et al., 2004; Skaper et al., 1998). A mechanism likely underlying the effects of melatonin on synaptic plasticity is a modulation of the intrinsic excitability of hippocampal neurons. Hyperpolarizaton induced by melatonin could reduce LTP by inhibiting NMDA receptor activation during high frequency stimulation (Wang et al., 2005). Melatonin application decreases membrane excitability in other regions of the nervous system in part via an enhancement of potassium currents (Wang et al., 2005). Melatonin also may decrease spontaneous action potential generation in the SCN (Shibata, Cassone, and Moore, 1989; Stehle, Vanecek, and Vollrath, 1989; Mason and Rusak, 1990) through an increase in a potassium conductance and a decrease in a hyperpolarization-activated current (Jiang et al., 1995; van den Top et al., 2001). Melatonin may also inhibit LTP induction through a regulation of signaling pathways downstream of the membrane and NMDA receptor activation and outside of the hippocampus, melatonin may influence rhythms in gene expression and second messenger systems (von Gall et al., 2002; Gerdin et al., 2004; Wang et al., 2005). Electrophysiological studies also have reported that melatonin may regulate the electrical activity of hippocampal neurons (Zeise and Semm, 1985; Musshoff et al., 2002) and alter synaptic transmission between hippocampal neurons (Wan et al., 1999; Hogan et al., 2001; El-Sherif et al., 2002). These findings indicate that melatonin can regulate learning and memory through its influence to synaptic connections within the hippocampus undergoing activity-dependent changes in synaptic strength including enhancements in the strength of excitatory synaptic transmission that regulates LTP.

In this context there is evidence that stress disrupts normal activity and memory consolidation in the hippocampus and prefrontal cortex (Diamond and Rose, 1994; Ruel and de Kloet, 1985; Payne et al., 2006; Bob and Fedor-Freybergh, 2008). This process leads to memories that are stored without a contextual or spatiotemporal frame and produce memories that are often fragmentary, temporally and spatially disorganized, mainly because they originate from entirely unrelated events. Disturbed temporal memory related to stress conditions is evident from studies focused on episodic and autobiographical memories and shows temporal disorganization, fragmentation and incompleteness but not necessary absence of emotion or dissociative amnesia (Kenardy et al., 2007; Payne et al., 2006; Brewin, 2007).

According to recent experimental findings stress-related events are related to melatonin alterations in animals and also in humans. For example, repeated maternal separation and deprivation caused low blood melatonin levels and a significant negative correlation between blood melatonin levels and spatial memory performance in both of male and female adolescent rats that suggest an association between melatonin production and neurodevelopment. (Uysal et al., 2005). Further studies also found the interaction between stress and pineal gland (Simonneaux and Ribelayga, 2003). Electron microscopy studies have found that immobilization stress induces pinealocyte degeneration (Milin, Demajo, and Todorovic, 1996). These alterations were related with significant increase of melatonin in rat pineal gland (Vollrath and Welker, 1998). Psychosocial stress also induced a robust increase of melatonin metabolite 6-sulfatoxymelatonin in subordinate animals (Fuchs and Schumacher, 1990), while in humans, sleep disturbances, such as insomnia (Jindal and Thase, 2004), and reduced nocturnal peak of pineal melatonin secretion that is often present in depressed patients (Brown et al., 1985; Frazer et al., 1986; Pacchierotti et al., 2001). These studies suggest that the pineal gland may be significantly affected by stress that is consistent with findings that pineal gland expresses high density of the glucocorticoid receptor (Warembourg, 1975; Sarrieau et al., 1988; Meyer et al., 1998). Melatonin receptors are also present in regions that participate in the stress response, such as the hippocampus or the adrenal gland (Musshoff et al., 2002; Torres-Farfan et al., 2003).

Together these findings suggest that melatonin likely is significantly associated with the regulation of memory, cognition and emotional processes (Laudon, Hyde, and Ben-Jonathan, 1989; Boatright, Rubim, and Iuvone, 1994; Hemby, Trojanowski, and Ginsberg, 2003). These findings emphasizing a specific role of melatonin in mechanisms of cognition, memory and stress are also consistent with reported studies that indicate melatonin alterations in psychopathology mainly in patients with depression, schizophrenia, anxiety disorders, eating disorders and also in other mental disorders (Pacchierotti et al., 2001; Bob and Fedor-Freybergh, 2008).

4.4. BRAIN DERIVED NEUROTROPHIC FACTOR (BDNF), TRAUMATIC STRESS AND DEPRESSION

BDNF is a polypeptide growth factor that influences differentiation and survival of neurons in the nervous system that is important in regulating synaptic plasticity and connectivity in the CNS with implications for mechanisms of memory storage and mood control (Bath and Lee, 2006; Bramham and Messaoudi, 2005). BDNF is an activity-dependent modulator of excitatory transmission and synaptic plasticity with predominant effective localization of BDNF and its receptor tyrosine kinase TrkB (tropomyosin receptor kinase B) on glutamate synapses (Soule, Messaoudi, and Bramham, 2006; Bramham and Messaoudi, 2005). Recent evidence indicates that endogenous BDNF-TrkB signaling in synaptic consolidation by long-term potentiation (LTP) needs new gene expression and protein synthesis that enables immediate early gene Arc (activity-regulated cytoskeleton-associated protein) (Bath and Lee, 2006; Bramham and Messaoudi, 2005; Soule, Messaoudi, and Bramham, 2006). Important factor in this new gene expression is also the transcription factor CREB, which is required for hippocampus-dependent long term memory formation (Mizuno and Giese, 2005). The CREB is activated by signaling pathways that include

Ca(2+)/calmodulin kinases (CaMKs), protein kinase A (PKA) and the mitogen activated protein/extracellular signal-regulated kinases (MAPK or ERKs) (Mizuno and Giese, 2005; Rattiner, Davis, and Ressler, 2005). Recent molecular genetic and behavioral studies also demonstrate that spatial and contextual types of hippocampus-dependent formation of long term memory require different signaling molecules implicating distinct types of hippocampus-dependent long term memory that differ in their underlying molecular mechanisms (Mizuno and Giese, 2005). As a part of these signaling pathways a basic mechanism of BDNF is that it may modulate both excitatory and inhibitory neurotransmitter systems (Savitz, Solms, and Ramesar, 2006). According to several studies BDNF also influences functions of serotonergic and dopaminergic systems (Savitz, Solms, and Ramesar, 2006; Narita et al., 2003; Mossner et al., 2000).

Relationship between BDNF and cognition is also mediated by influence of stress (Savitz, Solms, and Ramesar, 2006) because especially chronic stress influences excessive release of glucocorticoids from the adrenal gland that cause cell death or atrophy of vulnerable neurons through the cortisol action and inhibitory influence on BDNF synthesis in the hippocampus (Savitz, Solms, and Ramesar, 2006). Together recent findings suggest that BDNF may play an important role in stress response and related modification of synaptic plasticity, transmission and memory formation especially in the hippocampus and neocortex, and it has a specific role in depression, schizophrenia, epilepsy, neurodegenerative disorders and pain sensitization (Binder and Scharfman, 2004; Thomas and Davis, 2005).

These findings suggest that specific memory impairment in depression could be reflected in BDNF activity and that the typical BDNF changes in various regions of the CNS related to traumatic stress in pathogenesis of depression may occur. In principle, these data are consistent with reported relationship between dissociation and traumatic memories that has been found also in studies of depressive patients. According to Beck's cognitive theory of depression (Beck et al., 1979, 1996) many aspects of depressive cognition reflect the fact that the individual predominantly cannot recall negative past episodes. It is linked to activation of generalized schemas that consist of negative information about the self and activate specific less accessible autobiographical memories. A study reported by Spenceley and Jerom (1997), suggests that defensive reaction which leads to effort to eliminate these negative memories increases intrusive thoughts. Also other recent studies indicate that intrusive memories have an important role in depression (Brewin and Andrews, 1998; Wheatley et al., 2007; Patel et al., 2007). It implicates that the effort to avoid bad experiences paradoxically may increase their accessibility to the consciousness (Wegner, 1994). According to information-processing theories of depression, the greater accessibility of negative memories should lead to more severe and prolonged depression and predict it (Brewin and Andrews, 1998). Kuyken and Brewin (1995) reported close relationship between intrusive autobiographical memories of childhood abuse and other aspects of depressive cognition.

In addition, depressive patients (although less than PTSD patients) experience very vivid and distressing memories (Brewin and Andrews, 1998; Wheatley et al., 2007; Patel et al., 2007). The majority of the memories are accompanied by feelings and physical sensations reliving a traumatic event and represent dissociated fragments separated from normal mental phenomena. These depression related memory disturbances were also confirmed by relationship between dissociative and depressive symptoms in patients with depressive disorder (Wilkeson et al., 2000; Maaranen et al., 2005; Bob et al., 2005).

Chapter 5

PAIN, DISSOCIATION AND SUBLIMINAL CONSCIOUSNESS

5.1. PAIN AND CONSCIOUSNESS

Pain is a multidimensional experience that includes discriminative, affective, motivational and cognitive components mediated by spinal, brainstem, and cerebral functioning, modulated through forebrain mechanisms. Modern advances in pain research show that processing of painful experiences is based on widely distributed processing in the brain that is closely related to mechanisms of consciousness (Coghill et al., 1999; Price, Barrel and Rainville, 2002; Chen, 2001; Bob, 2008). Pain is defined as unpleasant sensory and emotional experience associated with actual or potential tissue damage, or described in terms of such damage (International Association for the Study of Pain Task Force on Taxonomy, 1994, p. 210). This definition implicates that pain represents unique sensory, perceptual and emotional characteristics related to state of consciousness. It necessarily leads to distinguishing between pain and nociception because there is a lack of absolute correspondence between pain and tissue damage (Eccleston and Crombez, 1999; Chapman and Nakamura 1999; Craig, 2003).

Pain is closely related to consciousness as emphasized by definition and there is also evidence that pain experiences may be modulated by cognition (Coghill et al., 1999; Villemure and Bushnell, 2002; Eccleston and Crombez, 1999; Tiengo, 2003). There are many pharmacological mechanisms in modulation of pain, but also psychological mechanisms such as attentiveness, emotional context, individual attitudes or personal expectations can influence experience of pain. These modulatory mechanisms can have analgesic or an anesthetic effect and alter the perception and transmission of nociceptive information. Important attribute represents also a way of cognition and perceiving environment that substantially changes experience of pain. Psychological factors that significantly influence pain modulation are attention and emotion (Coghill et al., 1999; Villemure and Bushnell, 2002; Eccleston and Crombez, 1999; Tiengo, 2003; Bob, 2008). A number of reports show that pain is perceived as less intense when individuals draw their attention away from the pain whereas focusing on pain enhances the pain experience. These findings are in accordance with evidence in humans and non-human primates that neuronal responsiveness in primary somatosensory cortices to non-painful as well as painful stimuli is altered by the degree of attention. These data are also in agreement with psychological findings about analgesia or anesthesia induced by hypnosis indicating that effectiveness of hypnotic analgesia of anesthesia varies with attention (Coghill et al., 1999; Villemure and Bushnell, 2002; Eccleston and Crombez, 1999; Petrovic and Ingvar, 2002).

Recent studies of attentional modulation of pain are in accordance with information processing models that attempt to describe attention as a filter, as a resource, and as a mechanism for response selection (Eccleston and Crombez, 1999). Attention is, from this point of view, defined as selection among potential conscious contents, characterized by global distribution of information (Baars, 1988, 2002). Function of attentional mechanism with respect to pain signals is to select the stimulus and bring different pain events into the consciousness. This novel painful stimulus will elicit an attentional shift, particularly after pain onset (Eccleston and Crombez, 1999). From this point of view, pain is understood as a warning signal to an organism from natural or social environment that interrupts, distracts, and demands attention (Eccleston and Crombez, 1999; Craig, 2003; Villemure, Slotnick, and Bushnell, 2003). In this context, there is increased understanding of higher cortical functions contribution to endogenous pain control. Pain interferes with concurrent activities and higher cortical functions may constitute a way of resolving cognitive and behavioral conflict by allowing competing task relevant stimuli to dominate over the pain (Eccleston and Crombez, 1999; Lorenz, Minoshima, and Casey, 2003; Bob, 2008). Various studies describe activity of prefrontal regions in clinical and experimental pain conditions (Silverman et al., 1997; Baron et al., 1999; Tolle et al., 1999; Lorenz et al., 2002; Bornhovd et al., 2002; Lorenz, Minoshima, and Casey, 2003; Bob, 2008). There is also evidence that medial prefrontal regions and the perigenual anterior cingulate cortex are activated by anticipation of pain, interaction of pain with anxiety, placebo conditions and other cognitively demanding tasks (Sawamoto et al., 2000; Ploghaus et al., 2001; Petrovic et al., 2002; Bantick et al., 2002; Lorenz, Minoshima, and Casey, 2003; Wager et al., 2004). Lorenz et al. (2003) reported that ratings of pain intensity and negative affect during heat allodynia (response to a normally warm stimulus on sensitized skin after capsaicin treatment) correlated negatively with activities in the right and left dorsolateral prefrontal cortex (DLPFC). The inter-regional correlation of midbrain and medial thalamic activity was significantly reduced during high left DLPFC activity.

The findings suggest that negative correlation of the left DLPFC activity with pain affect may relate to decreased effective connectivity (i.e. flow of neural information) of the midbrain-medial thalamic pathway. In contrast, increased right DLPFC activity relates to weakened relationship of the anterior insula with both pain intensity and affect (Lorenz, Minoshima, and Casey, 2003). These findings are consistent with invasive studies performed in animals, for example, Hardy and Haigler (1985) reported that electrical stimulation of the prefrontal cortex depressed the midbrain response to noxious stimuli in rats. Similar suppression found Andersen (1986) in the medial thalamic response to noxious stimuli caused by electrical stimulation of the periaqueductal grey matter or the frontal (pericruciate) cortex in cats. In addition, the existence of a pain modulation pathway involving the midbrain, medial thalamus and prefrontal cortex in rodents has been reported (Condes-Lara et al., 1989). Functional dissociation within the midbrain may therefore enable facilitatory as well as inhibitory influence on pain and affect (Hirakawa et al., 2000). Reported positive correlation of the ventral/orbitofrontal cortex (VOFC) activity and pain (Lorenz, Minoshima, and Casey, 2003) is in accordance with findings that show increased activity of these regions during expectation of pain and its exacerbation by anxiety (Lorenz, Minoshima, and Casey, 2003; Sawamoto et al., 2000; Ploghaus et al., 2001; Bob, 2008).

A role of DLPFC in the control of nociceptive information is confirmed by findings that show this region as closely associated with efficient performance in the presence of conflicting stimuli (MacDonald et al., 2000; Bunge et al., 2001). For example, working memory task related to keeping information in the mind requires a high degree of executive control that is typically associated with high DLPFC activity (Smith and Ionides, 1999; Funahashi, 2001). Functional dissociation of DLPFC may protect maintenance of momentary behavioral goals by rendering working memory operations resistant to distractive stimuli (Sakai et al., 2002). In contrast to DLPFC, ventrolateral PFC may play a greater role in filtering out irrelevant information and selecting among competing stimuli, responses and associations (Thompson-Schill et al., 1997; Jonides et al., 1998; Hazeltine et al., 2000; Leung et al., 2000; Bunge et al., 2001). On the other hand, higher activation of anterior cingulate is related to detecting cognitive conflict and signaling the need for greater allocation of attention for the purpose of resolving conflict (MacDonald et al., 2000; Bunge et al., 2001; Oschner et al., 2001; Raz, Fan, and Posner, 2005; Egner, Jamieson, and Gruzelier, 2005). Taken together, these findings suggest that the anterior cingulate is involved in detecting conflict and that lateral PFC is involved in resolving the conflict (Bunge et al., 2001). Recent findings show that specific hypnotic suggestions also reduce involuntary conflict and alter information processes in highly hypnotizable individuals. According to fMRI results highly hypnotizable persons under hypnotic suggestion show reduced ACC activity in comparison with either no-suggestion or less hypnotizable controls (Raz, Fan, and Posner, 2005).

5.2. Hypnosis, Pain and Divided Consciousness

Concept of attentional filtering in nociceptive information processing is consistent with research findings expanding and evolving neurophysiological model of hypnosis. This concept supports the view, that highly hypnotizable persons posses stronger attentional filtering abilities than low hypnotizable and that these differences are reflected in underlying brain dynamics such as an interplay between cortical and subcortical structures (Eccleston and Crombez, 1999, Crawford, 1994; Feldman, 2004; Bob, 2008). Highly hypnotizable persons can better focus and sustain their attention as well as better ignore irrelevant stimuli from the environment (Crawford, 1994). It corresponds to findings that descending inhibitory pathways, parallel to ascending sensory systems can modulate quite early responses related to sensory information. This suggests that high hypnotizables can better inhibit incoming sensory stimuli and it is in accordance with recent models of attention, which propose that the frontal cortex regulates the limbic system in the active gating of incoming sensory stimuli (Crawford, 1994). Consequently, the attentional shift because of a pain stimulus is linked to characteristic changes of neural activity patterns or "neurosignature" patterns of nerve impulses generated by a widely distributed neural network- the "body-self neuromatrix"- in the brain (Melzack, 1999, 2001).

Modulation of attention in hypnotic states is coupled to the global changes in subjective experience and markedly influences regulation and monitoring body and mental state, experiencing of the self and underlying process of self-representation. Self-representation as a mental structure creating identity and awareness can be defined as a result of interpretation of certain inner states of own body as parts of mental and somatic identity, while other bodily signals are interpreted as perceptions of the external world. Alterations in "self-representation" that underly the changes in subjective experience are linked to a great and abrupt changes in patterns of neural activity. This supports the notion that hypnosis, because of significant attentional shift, leads to a distinct "state" of consciousness (Rainville et al., 1997, 2002; Metzinger, 2000). Another way of looking at the hypnotic lack of the self-representation can be observed as dissociated or divided consciousness (Crawford, 1994; Hilgard, 1986; Vermetten and Bremner, 2004; Bob, 2008).

In clinical studies these hypnotic alterations of consciousness have been found as suitable methods for cognitive modulation of painful experience. These data show that hypnosis modulates activity in brain structures involved in the regulation of consciousness and enables to perform analgesia or anesthesia in many individuals (Rainville et al., 1997; Rainville et al., 2002). Recent findings confirm the influence of hypnosis on decreased sensitivity to pain in well-controlled experiments (Montgomery, DuHamel, and Redd, 2000; Lynn et al., 2000; Patterson and Jensen, 2003; Jensen and Patterson, 2005). For example, Patterson and Jensen (2003) reviewed the number of controlled clinical studies and found conclusive arguments that hypnotic analgesia is associated with significant reduction of subjective pain ratings, decreased need for analgesics or sedation, lower occurrence of nausea and vomiting, and decreased length of hospitalization. Hypnotic treatment is also associated with better overall outcome after hospitalization and greater physiological stability. They concluded that hypnotic techniques for the relief of acute pain as an outcome of tissue damage are superior to standard care and often better than other methods of pain treatment, and that hypnosis has a reliable and significant impact on acute procedural pain, and chronic pain conditions (Patterson and Jensen, 2003). Similarly, a meta-analytic study published by Montgomery et al. (2000) showed that 75% of clinical and experimental participants with different types of pain obtained substantial pain relief from hypnotic techniques. This implicates that hypnosis is effective for most people suffering from diverse forms of pain with the exception of minority of patients resistant to hypnotic therapy. Reported studies show a moderate to large hypnoanalgesic effect that confirm efficacy of hypnotic techniques for pain management. The findings indicate that hypnotic suggestion was equally effective in reducing both clinical and experimental pain. The overall results suggest broader application of hypnoanalgesic techniques with pain patients (Montgomery et al., 2000; Jensen et al., 2006; Elkins et al., 2006; Patterson, Wiechman, Jensen, and Sharar, 2006; Elkins, Jensen, and Patterson, 2007; Hammond, 2007).

In this context recent results also show that hypnosis may specifically influence both pain unpleasantness and pain intensity. For example, Rainville et al. (1997, 1999) found significant relationship between pain unpleasantness and ACC pain-evoked activity after hypnotic suggestions. The results strongly indicate the involvement of ACC in the affective dimension of the pain experience, consistently with results of lesion studies suggesting that post-cingulotomy patients show a reduction in pain related emotional responses (Rainville et al. 1997; Corkin and Hebben 1981; Foltz and Lowell, 1962; Foltz and White, 1968). On the other hand, hypnotic suggestions directed toward pain sensation produced significant changes in somatosensory cortex S1 (with a similar trend in S2 cortex) but not in the ACC (Hofbauer et al., 2001). These findings show that structures of cerebral nociceptive network including subcortical regions, such as thalamus, basal ganglia, insular region, limbic circuits, ACC and somatosensory regions S1 and S2 may contribute differentially to the pain experience although the anatomical connections among these structures suggest that these regions do not function independently in encoding of different aspects of pain experience. These data show that attentional modulation and selection related to hypnotic dissociation may determine not only pain reinterpretation but also pain reduction that is consistent with influence of hypnosis on somatosensory perception (Spiegel, 2003; Spiegel et al., 1989; Kosslyn et al. 2000; Bob, 2008).

5.3. PAIN AND DISSOCIATION

Similar conditions that lead to the modulation of pain in hypnosis occur also in cases of traumatic dissociation. In these states instead of hypnosis a frightening experience may cause the attentional shift to a mental state that does not fit into existing cognitive schemes and memories of the frightening experience are split off (or dissociated) from consciousness (van der Kolk and van der Hart, 1989; Bob, 2008). This shift between self-representations is linked to typical attention-induced changes of neural patterns and every self-representation is mediated by multiple processing of inner stimuli on different levels of the CNS. Multiple processing at different levels leads to re-representations of the interoceptive images of the physiological condition of the material body, which include also pain stimuli. These re-representations on the level of interoceptive cortex, linked to a meta-representation of the state of the body, are probably functionally associated in the field of right anterior insula which is linked to subjective awareness of the 'feeling self'. Pain from this point of view represents a specific somatic distress signal that is integrated within the contexts of current physiological and environmental conditions and past experience (Craig, 2001, 2002, 2003).

Dissociation is defined as a disturbance or alteration of normal integrated functions of consciousness, memory or identity that leads also to characteristic somatoform changes (Hall and Powell, 2000; Putnam, 1989; van der Kolk and van der Hart, 1989; Nijenhuis et al., 1996, 2000; Bob 2003a, 2008). Somatoform dissociation as a lack of integration of somatoform components of experience, reactions and functions represents alterations in sensation of pain (analgesia, kinesthetic anesthesia), painful symptoms, alterations of perception, motor inhibition, loss of motor control, gastrointestinal symptoms and other (Nijenhuis et al., 1996; Nijenhuis, 2000). Dissociation on the psychic level emerges as memory losses, fragmentation of knowledge of the self and experience, splitting of emotional and/or cognitive aspects of experiences, numbing of affect, psychological escape from unpleasant stimuli, trance-like states, increased suggestibility and greater hypnotizability (Putnam, 1989, 1997; Hall and Powell, 2000; van der Kolk and van der Hart, 1989).

Dissociation in most cases occurs due to a traumatic event. Most often, this event represents exposition of a trauma in childhood because of physical, emotional or sexual abuse with following development of symptoms often after many years. Dissociative symptoms also occur due to traumatic events such as accidents, nature calamities etc. Characteristic features of psychic dissociative symptoms are changes in notion of personal identity as depersonalization or in serious cases may develop multiple personality disorder characterized by distinguished personalities that exist in one person. Other experienced symptoms represent changes in notion of external world such as derealization, hallucinations or changes of memory, for example psychogenic amnesia or multiple personality (Putnam, 1989; Hall and Powell, 2000; Spiegel and Cardena, 1991; Vermetten and Bremner, 2004; Bob, 2008). In multiple personality disorder the patients manifest two or more distinct identities or personality states that recurrently take control of behavior and consciousness (Putnam, 1989, 1997). Extremely stressful and traumatic conditions may cause switching within a spectrum of self-reference frames. At this point multiple personality disorder is most complex form of dissociation related to a loss of adaptive form of self-awareness and identity. Multiple personality disorder can be understood as an extreme form of shame and conformity caused by social pressure that determine denial of certain own feelings, ideas, patterns of behavior and resulting identity as a form of switching self-reference. These fluctuating states of consciousness and self-awareness within one human brain represent a form of personality-state-dependent information processing. Their typical manifestation in the brain areas and networks involved in experience of the self was reported by neuroimaging data (Reinders et al., 2003). Typical problem regarding multiple personality disorder represents non-realistic fantasy linked to this disease that obscures its understanding and diagnostics in usual context of dissociative disorders.

5.4. DISSOCIATION AND PAIN THRESHOLD

Relationship between dissociation and pain threshold was documented in many studies that reported effects similar to modulation of pain in hypnosis. Because of many similarities with hypnosis, pathological dissociative states are sometimes called hypnoid states because of possible "autohypnotic process" (Frankel, 1996; Hilgard, 1986; Butler et al., 1996). In this context several studies indicate that some victims of a traumatic experience are unable to register pain (for example during self-injury) or painful affects (Butler et al., 1996; Frankel, 1996; Agargun et al., 1998; Ebrinc, 2002; Trief, 1996; Saxe, Chawla and van der Kolk, 2002; Russr et al., 1993; Orbach et al., 1997). Patients with dissociative disorders also frequently report amnesia for self-injury (Saxe, Chawla and van der Kolk, 2002; Putnam, 1989). These changes in pain perception similarly as in hypnosis are probably a consequence of profound changes in affect state, memory and sense of identity in response to environmental stress injury (Saxe, Chawla and van der Kolk, 2002). These profound changes also lead to the lack of the self-representation and are related to changes in patterns of neural activity (Crawford, 1994; Vermetten and Bremner, 2004). In these conditions, significant changes in interpretation of inner signals also occur and this novel interpretation has consequences for sensing of own identity and external world. According to Helen Watkins' concept (Watkins,

1993) these dissociated self-representations emerge as ego states (or hidden observers even in non-multiple subjects) and represent organized cognitive structural system of segments of the personality often similar to true multiple personalities. These dissociated self-representations were also reported in normal people in hypnosis and during dreaming in subjects with multiple personality disorder (Watkins and Watkins, 1979-80; Bowers and Brecher, 1955; Watkins, 1993; Lynn et al., 1994; Merskey, 1992; Rickeport, 1992; Barret, 1995, 1996).

An ability to describe unconsciously perceived pain was also reported in cases of multiple personality where similar entity as the hidden observer called internal self–helper was found (Alison, 1974; Putnam, 1989; Saley, 1988). According to these studies, internal self-helper may know other personalities dissolved by amnestic barrier and their organization and relationships. In therapeutic practice, the internal self-helper may become the center of the treatment for the integration of the personality (Alison, 1974; Putnam, 1989; Saley, 1988; Gabel, 1989; Bob, 2004) and similarly as the hidden observer in hypnosis is able to recover traumatic and painful accidents (Watkins and Watkins, 1979-80; Watkins, 1993; Lynn et al., 1994; Bob, 2008). The internal self-helper similarly as the hidden observer may represent subliminally stored memories that likely include also self-related functions. From this point of view, dissociated painful experience remains a part of cognitive and behavioral strategies that indirectly influence consciousness (Bob, 2008).

5.5. RELATIONSHIP BETWEEN PAIN AND DISSOCIATION

According to above reviewed findings there is partial supportive evidence for the hypothesis that hypnotically or trauma induced dissociative states can lead to inability to perceive emotional or physical pain. Several findings also suggest that this painful information in certain cases may be recalled later. In these occasions, dissociative state probably acts as a defense mechanism that raises pain threshold due to intended hypnotic modulation or threatened life situation that induces dissociation. A relationship between physical pain and dissociation is also reported in pain medicine in cases of chronic pain associated with following dissociative symptoms or dissociative disorders (Fishbain et al., 2001). Several studies suggest that patients with chronic pelvic pain were significantly more likely to use dissociation as a coping mechanism and significantly more likely experienced severe childhood sexual abuse (Walker et al., 1992; Badura et al., 1997). Other studies reported significant occurrence of memory disturbances in the patients with chronic pain (Luoto et al., 1999; Iezzi et al., 1999). Similar association between chronic physical pain and dissociation has also been described in patients with dissociative disorders such as multiple personality disorder (Frances and Spiegel, 1987; Livengood et al., 1994; McFadden and Woitalla, 1993; McFadden, 1992; Fishbain et al., 2001; Bob, 2008). For example, a 34-year-old woman with chronic pain of the right wrist who developed multiple personality disorder (Frances and Spiegel, 1987) or a male who demonstrated another personality during the period of a severe untreated headache (Livengood et al., 1994). Conversely, a most common somatic complaint in patients with multiple personality disorder headaches were reported (Greaves, 1980; Bliss, 1980; Coons, Bowman and Milstein,1988; Coons et al., 1988; Coons, 1980; Putnam et al., 1986). Symptoms of headaches in multiple personality disorder patients have been described as extremely painful during the switching of personalities (Coons Coons, Bowman and Milstein,1988; Coons, 1980; Larmore et al., 1977; Packard and Brown, 1986). Several reported cases also suggest that multiple personality disorder patients can eliminate pain in the primary personality by displacing it into other alters (Watkins and Watkins, 1990). Serious symptoms of headaches have also been reported in association with a sudden unexpected travel away with amnesia and confusion about personal identity in patients with dissociative fugue (O'Brien, 1985; Fishbain et al., 2001).

On the other hand, recent findings suggest the possibility that an experience of pain can originate exclusively within a subject's brain or mind rather than being necessarily dependent on the pathology of peripheral tissue (Derbyshire et al., 2004). The existence of a neural functional pain mechanism support findings that specific modulation of brain activity enables manipulation of affective and sensory dimensions of pain experience (Coghill et al., 2003; Croft, 2000; Derbyshire et al., 1994, 1997, 2002; Faymonville et al., 2003; Gracely et al., 2002; Rainville et al., 1997; Bob, 2008).

For example, abnormal activation within the pain network has been postulated to cause or partially generate certain clinical pain disorders such as chronic low back pain, atypical facial pain, and fibromyalgia (Derbyshire et al., 1994, 2002; Gracely et al., 2002). These disorders belong to the group of functional pain disorders, defined as consisting of one or more symptoms that, after appropriate medical assessment, cannot be explained in terms of a conventionally defined medical disease (Wessely et al., 1999).

Recent findings also show close relationship between pain and detecting cognitive conflict in the anterior cingulate that implicates interconnection of stress, negative affect, and pain. These data suggest that various stimuli ranging from injury elsewhere in the body as well as emotional and cognitive inputs from higher neural centers can expand, amplify, or create pain symptoms (Croft, 2000; Derbyshire, 2004).

As mentioned above, recent findings show that specific hypnotic suggestion reduces involuntary conflict and alters information processes in highly hypnotizable individuals. The fMRI results also revealed reduced ACC activity under hypnotic suggestion in highly hypnotizable persons compared with either no-suggestion or less hypnotizable controls (Raz, Fan, and Posner, 2005). On the other hand hypnotic suggestion may likely cause enhanced ACC activity that can be experienced as pain, as suggest fMRI data obtained during conditions of physically and hypnotically induced experiences of heat pain interleaved with periods of rest that revealed common activation of the thalamus, ACC, midanterior insula, and parietal and prefrontal cortices (Derbyshire et al., 2004). These findings demonstrate the efficacy of suggestion following hypnotic induction similarly as in cases in which hypnotic suggestion produced altered sensory experience with specificity of the response to the stimulus (Faymonville et al., 2003; Rainville et al., 1997; Bob, 2008). In comparison to the rest condition, the experimental conditions show that both pain from a nociceptive source and hypnotically induced pain activate regions of the brain that have been described as belonging to a pain neuromatrix (Casey, 1999; Derbyshire, 2000; Peyron et al., 2000; Price, 2000; Treede et al., 1999). These results support a successive-stage model of pain processing in which pain unpleasantness is highly but not exclusively dependent on pain sensations. The present clinical data indicate that deficits in pain sensations after lesions to somatosensory cortices S1 and S2 may cause absence of a painful sensation after pain stimulus although the patient may experience ill-localized and ill-defined unpleasant feeling in the absence of a clear pain sensation (Greenspan et al. 1999; Hofbauer et al., 2001; Ploner et al. 1999). These data illustrate that dissociated sensations may produce pain affect in the absence of pain sensation (Hofbauer et al., 2001). Similar mechanism likely may be used in hypnotic or traumatic dissociation that may cause differential activation of regions belonging to pain network that produce specific affective and sensory pain experiences. With respect to connectivity of the ACC with DLPFC it is possible that the ACC facilitate the integration and interpretation of sensory signals based on the expectations generated by the DLPFC and that the ACC may serve to regulate perceptions in relation to changes in cognition or motivational states (Goffaux et al., 2007; Paus, 2001).

These data strongly suggest that pain on various levels may be transformed and that experienced physical pain per se may contribute to manifestation of dissociative state. Pain experience induced by psychological traumatic stress as well as physical pain that leads to hopelessness and conflict incapable of sollution such as in cases of chronic pain probably may induce dissociation. Above reported data are in accordance with evidence, that dissociation may modulate pain and serves as a defense mechanism. In many reported cases of psychiatric patients, we can found mutual relationship between traumatic stress producing emotional pain and painful physical symptoms. Neurophysiological basis for this relationship may be established on higher activation of anterior cingulate that is characteristic for pain perception but it is also closely related to detecting cognitive conflict, which is undoubtedly characteristic for cognitive disintegration in dissociative states. It could be therefore possible that cognitive conflict may be represented as pain and on the other hand, physical pain mainly in chronic forms may lead to extreme cognitive conflict resulting to dissociation of cognitive components emerging as dissociative symptoms. This hypothesis is in accordance with findings that functional dissociation of the ventromedial/orbital and lateral prefrontal cortex has also been described in studies of abnormal brain chemistry in chronic pain patients (Grachev et al., 2000, 2002). This is consistent with findings that the functional dissociation of medial structures probably may enable facilitating as well as inhibitory influences on pain and affect (Hirakawa et al., 2000). These data support the view that both physical painful symptoms as well as dissociative symptoms, which are closely related to psychological pain, have common neurophysiological substrate associated with mechanisms of consciousness.

5.6. PAIN AND SOCIAL RELATIONSHIPS

These findings that constitute pain also as a psychological phenomenon are in accordance with experiencing of psychological pain where "nociception" represents traumatic stimuli from social environment even without direct or potential nociceptive stimulation (Bob, 2008). Although predominant view of international pain research community is that it does not distinguish between physical and emotional pain and regards these as metaphors, this view is not always sufficient in psychology and psychiatry. In psychological and psychiatric theory and practice we can find various cases of painful experiences, which do not confirm the definition that pain is unpleasant sensory and emotional experience associated with actual or potential tissue damage, or described in terms of such damage (International Association for the Study of Pain Task Force on Taxonomy, 1994, p. 210). A common phenomenon in psychological and psychiatric practice is a subjective pain experience caused by conditions related to goal directed behavior, social loss or frustration, which do not represent any direct potential tissue damage or threatening life situations. In this context, recent findings suggest that psychological pain related to social exclusion, social loss and empathy causes activation of certain human brain areas activated also during physical pain (Panksepp, 2003; Eisenberg, Lieberman, and Williams, 2003; Eisenberg and Lieberman, 2004; Singer et al., 2004; Bob, 2008). For example, during experiments related to feeling of social exclusion, fMRI measures show that subjects experienced emotional distress as indicated by substantial blood flow changes in two key brain regions. The first one was the anterior cingulate cortex that is also related to generating the aversive experience of physical pain. The second was the prefrontal cortex that displays an opposite activity pattern characterized by increased activation when the distress was weakened (Panksepp, 2003; Eisenberg, Lieberman, and Williams, 2003). Another example shows the study by Singer et al. (2004), who experimentally tested human ability to share an experience of another's pain as a function of empathy. They use functional imaging for the assessment of brain activity while volunteers experienced a painful stimulus and compared it to the activity elicited in situations when their loved one in the same room was receiving a similar pain stimulus. They found that bilateral anterior insula, rostral anterior cingulate cortex, brainstem, and cerebellum were activated immediately when subjects received pain stimuli or during the observation of loved ones suffering. The study also indicates that activations in anterior insula and ACC are significantly correlated with individual empathy scores. Activations in the posterior insula/secondary somatosensory cortex, the sensorimotor cortex and the caudal ACC were specific to pain experience. The data indicate that a neural substrate for empathic experience does not involve the entire "pain matrix". Only the part of the pain network associated with its affective qualities, but not its sensory qualities, mediates empathy (Singer et al., 2004). With respect to difference between psychological and physical pain these data suggest that intensive aversive feelings associated with 'psychological pain' share a certain common regions with physical pain. This coactivation in certain brain regions probably explains the common qualities of both phenomena (Panksepp, 2003; Eisenberg, Lieberman, and Williams, 2003; Eisenberg and Lieberman, 2004; Singer et al., 2004; Bob, 2008).

Taken together, these findings signify that the cortical representation of signals from the body, including pain, provide basis for human awareness of the physical self as a feeling entity. This association provides a fundamental framework for the involvement of these feelings with emotion, mood, motivation and consciousness, and degrees of conscious awareness related to successive upgrades in the self-representational maps (Craig, 2001, 2002, 2003).

5.6. PAIN AND PSYCHOTHERAPY

In this context research of pain experience in connection with hypnosis, traumatic dissociation and subliminal processes provides important data for the study of consciousness with important consequences for psychotherapy. In these conditions dissociative state acts as a defense mechanism that raises pain threshold due to intended hypnotic modulation or threatened life situation that induce dissociation (Butler, Duran, Jasiukaitis, Koopman, and Spiegel, 1996; Frankel, 1996; Agargun, Tekeoglu, Kara, Adak, Ercan, 1998). From this point of view the hidden observer reflects the fact that dissociation between dominant conscious state and other states is not complete and there is meta-interpreter level which reflects different levels of interpretation and creates the base for integrity of consciousness. This is in accordance with understanding of consciousness as a gateway to brain integration that enables access between otherwise separated neuronal functions (Baars, 2002). This hypothesis also corresponds to known clinical evidence which shows that awareness, understanding and acceptance of the experienced traumatic event are able to treat dissociative symptoms and enables integration of dissociated painful memories.

These findings suggest that experience of pain in many cases plays an important role in human growth and spirituality, although it may be in contrast to hedonic aspect of our culture that tend to ignore painful experience as a part of human life. Recent research findings in posttraumatic growth strongly indicate that experience of pain can help to uncover real meaning of personal existence and that the self-reflection is an essential principle for the process of learning and creative understanding. In this context, in psychology and psychiatry is a long tradition to study the response to traumatic stress and its resolution that can enable positive personal changes although personal distress and growth may be coexisting (Yalom and Lieberman, 1991; Cadell, Regehr, and Hemsworth, 2003; Tedeschi and Calhoun, 1996, 2004; Zoellner and Maercker, 2006; Bob, 2008). These positive changes often include improved relationships, new life possibilities, a greater appreciation of life and spiritual development. Posttraumatic growth have been reported in various conditions such as in people who experienced bereavement, cancer, HIV, heart attacks, rheumatoid arthritis, bone marrow transplantation, sexual abuse or combat and transportation accidents (Tedeschi and Calhoun, 1996, 2004; Calhoun and Tedeschi, 2004; Zoellner and Maercker, 2006). These data show that individuals who are facing to a trauma are more frequently cognitively engaged with fundamental existential questions about death and the purpose of life and a commonly reported change is ability of the individual to value the smaller things in life with frequent interest in spiritual growth, philosophy and religion (Tedeschi and Calhoun, 2004). More comprehensive study on the posttraumatic growth perspectives is therefore very useful for psychotherapy and stress management, and potentially presents important part of various clinical and research programs that can help in self-reflection and deeper understanding of the human mind.

5.7. Consciousness and the Self

Recent evidence from behavioral studies of normal subjects as well as neurological patients show that perceptual information can be represented in the mind/brain without the subject's awareness of that information (Fernandez-Duque, 2003; Mericle et al., 2001; Kihlstrom, 2004; Shevrin, 2001; Smith and Bulman-Fleming 2004). These data suggest that awareness of perceptual information requires not only a strong representation of the contents of awareness but also access to that information by other parts of the mind/brain (Baars, 1988, 2002). The idea that access to the relevant representations is a substantial constraint on perceptual awareness is in accordance with evidence in the brain-damaged patients. Damage may disrupt neural pathways and perceptual information represented in one neural structure is not accessed by other parts of the system. On the other hand, conscious access to perceptual information may also change over time even in undamaged brains (Kanwisher, 2001). According to conscious access hypothesis, consciousness might be a gateway to brain integration that may enable access between otherwise separated neuronal functions (Baars, 2002). There is evidence for a mutual dependence between consciousness and executive input in cases of executive dysfunctions in patients with multiple personality, dissociative fugue and also during hypnosis. In these cases was reported a loss of one executive interpreter's access to conscious events while another was dominant (Hilgard 1986; Putnam 1986, 1997; Baars, 2002). Binding between conscious contents and self-function observed in these cases constitutes the self-representational dimension of consciousness which is characterized by interpretation of certain inner states of own body as mental and somatic identity, while other bodily signals are interpreted as perceptions of the external world. Self-representations that are currently not accessible to the dominant interpreter's access are dissociated and may be defined as subliminal self-representations (Bob, 2008). These subliminal self-representations as dissociated subsystems have sensory, emotional and cognitive elements that may be misinterpreted and experienced as physical pain with affective or sensory dimension because it is not adequately attributed as recovered painful memory and expectation caused by conflicting and dangerous situation. This process of misinterpretation likely cause that physical and emotional pain can become confused and that one of them in a dissociated state may turn into the other. Similar situation may also occur during projection (or transference) when inner psychic states are interpreted as external parts of other persons or during hallucinations certain internally generated voices or images are interpreted as sensory signals from external world (Feinberg, 1978; Feinberg and Guazzelli, 1999; Ford et al., 2001; Tsakiris et al., 2005). These data suggest that self-recognition is a specific cognitive process typically involving conscious experience and interpretation activity. Disruptions of these interpretation processes likely represent a neurophysiological substrate for the process of fragmentation of consciousness because of misattribution of certain inner states that may be interpreted as painful bodily signals or external objects because they are disowned and dissociated from consciousness. Psychological or physical pain stimuli leading to hopelessness and conflicting situation without known solution are "unacceptable", i.e. do not fit into current cognitive scheme because of dissociation, which may lead to "depersonalization" of certain emotions and cognitive strategies that create discrete "ego-states" or alter-personalities in multiple personality disorder divided from predominant state of consciousness (Bob, 2008).

From this point of view the hidden observer or internal self-helper in multiple personality reflect the fact that dissociation between dominant conscious state and other states is not complete and there is a meta-interpreter level which reflects different levels of interpretation and creates the base for integrity of consciousness. This is in accordance with understanding of consciousness as a gateway to brain integration that enables access between otherwise separated neuronal functions (Baars, 2002). This hypothesis also corresponds to known clinical evidence which shows that awareness, understanding and acceptation of the experienced traumatic event are able to treat dissociative symptoms and enable integration of dissociated painful memories.

Chapter 6

DISSOCIATION AND DREAMING BRAIN

6.1. THE MULTIPLE PERSONALITY AS A MODEL OF THE DISSOCIATED CHARACTER OF THE HUMAN PSYCHE AND MODEL FOR DREAMING

In multiple personality disorder the patients manifest two or more distinct identities or personality states that recurrently take control of behavior and consciousness (Putnam, 1989, 1997). Etiologically it is related to extremely stressful and traumatic conditions that may cause defense behavior which manifests as switching within a spectrum of self-reference frames that present as distinguished identities. At this point multiple personality disorder is a most complex form of dissociation related to a loss of adaptive form of self-awareness and identity. In this context multiple personality disorder can be understood as an extreme form of shame and conformity caused by social pressure that determine denial of certain own feelings, ideas, patterns of behavior and resulting disrupted identity in a form of switching self-reference and identity. These fluctuating states of consciousness and self-awareness within one human brain represent a form of personality-state-dependent information processing.

In the 1980 DSM III (Diagnostic and Statistical Manual of Mental Disorders) (American Psychiatric Association, 1987), the criteria of the multiple personality were introduced for the first time. The revised classification criteria for multiple personality (i.e. dissociative identity disorder) according to DSM IV are follows (American Psychiatric Association, 1994):

1. The presence of two or more distinct identities or personality states (each with its own relatively enduring pattern of perceiving, relating to, and thinking about the environment and self).
2. At least two of these identities or personality states recurrently take control of the person's behavior.
3. Inability to recall important personal information that is too extensive to be explained by ordinary forgetfulness.

4. The disturbance is not due to the direct physiological effects of a substance (e.g.,
    blackouts or chaotic behavior during Alcohol Intoxication) or a general medical
    condition (e.g., complex partial seizures).

Note: In children, the symptoms are not attributable to imaginary playmates or other
fantasy play.

   According to traditional concepts the personality becomes alternating and dissociated as
a consequence of splitting which cause that several personalities are distinguishable in one
person (Boleloucky, 1986; Bob, 2004; Bleuler, 1924). Typical structure may include birth
personality and a set of host personalities. The birth personality develops in the individual
from birth, while the personality that controls the body for most of the time, analogical to the
ego-complex, is called the host personality. Birth and host personalities are called primary,
while other personalities are called secondary. The presenting personality is the one actually
present at a given moment. As a consequence of therapy or hypnotic suggestion, the
personalities may integrate or fuse. Occasionally, they may integrate spontaneously
(Boleloucky, 1986; Bob, 2004).

   In the past, the multiple personality disorder as a subject of study was grouped with
dissociative disorders, such as hysterical neurosis. In ICD 10 (World Health Organization,
1993), the multiple personality belongs to the group of dissociative disorders (F 44).
Extending the concept of schizophrenia was also considered by Bleuler among others. He
also felt that multiple personality disorder was a rare phenomenon of great theoretical value
(Boleloucky, 1986; Bob, 2004; Bleuler, 1924). Bleuler also defined schizophrenia as a
disorder of integrity and thought that schizophrenia produces different personalities (Bob,
2004; Bleuler, 1924; Rosenbaum, 1980; Bottero, 2001; Scharfetter, 1998). As Rosenbaum
(1980) reported, review of index medicus from 1903 to the revival of interest in multiple
personality in 1978 shows a dramatic decline in the number of reports of multiple personality,
which indicates that many patients with multiple personality had been diagnosed and treated
as schizophrenia patients (Rosenbaum, 1980). It corresponds to findings that a substantial
number of patients with multiple personality disorder have previous diagnoses of
schizophrenia (Bottero, 2001; Scharfetter, 1998). Likely it is mainly due to the presence of
positive symptoms of schizophrenia in patients with dissociative identity disorder that report
more positive symptoms of schizophrenia than patients with schizophrenia. It is important to
note that schizophrenic patients report more negative symptoms. A primary emphasis on
positive symptoms may result in false-positive diagnoses of schizophrenia and false-negative
diagnoses of dissociative identity disorder (Ellason and Ross, 1995). In this context
substantial data show that psychotic symptoms occur in patients with multiple personality
disorder (or dissociative identity disorder). This overlap occurs also in schizophrenia patients
who display significant level of traumatic stress and dissociation (Foote and Park, 2008).
Similar findings reported also other studies that examine dissociation in schizophrenic
patients (Bernstein and Putnam, 1986; Spitzer, Haug and Freyberger, 1997; Startup, 1999;
Read et al., 2001).

   The creation of personalities, according to Bleuler (Bob, 2004; Bleuler, 1924; Bottero,
2001; Scharfetter, 1998), is the same as the process of splitting in schizophrenia. Among its
characteristic symptoms belong the emergence of alter personalities and typical amnesia.
Etiology is thus traditionally explained along the lines of Pierre Janet (Janet, 1890; van der

Hart and Friedman, 1989; Bob, 2004; Putnam, 1989) as being a consequence of dissociative reaction, analogous to somnambulism, fugue states, hypnosis or psychogenic amnesia, most often as a consequence of abuse or traumatic experiences mainly occuring between the ages of four to eight. It is a splitting of psychic connections similar to hysteria, but in an extreme version. Psychotic decompensation of some personality may occur and has corresponding symptoms, such as hallucinations.

Because of a spontaneous course or therapy, elucidating information among secondary personalities, is possible. Nevertheless the host personality often does not have this knowledge. An Internal Self–helper repeatedly appears (Putnam, 1989; Allison, 1974) that has knowledge of other personalities and their organization and relationships. It often becomes the center of the treatment for the integration of the personality.

In hypnosis with healthy individuals a similar entity called the "hidden observer" can be also present (Hilgard, 1986). The hidden observer or internal Self-helper could empirically corresponds to Jung's the Self (das Selbst).

According to Jung (1972, 1972a), associated connections of dissociated fragments of the personality represent a certain psychic entity which he called the Self. According to him, compensating integration processes in cases of pathological dissociation lead to the generation of symbols of the Self that stand for the psychic wholeness. These symbols represent psychic contents that penetrate separated psychic structures. In the case of a multiple personality, it leads to the manifestation of the Internal Self-helper that has knowledge of other parts of the psyche and has the ability to integrate other alter personalities. The Self thus represents the wholeness of psychic processes manifested by way of dreams, fantasies or projections in the form of gods, people, animals, vegetables or objects. Dissociation is thus compensated by factors that create connections, relationships, and knowledge among these dissociated psychic structures.

Using the perspective of the complex theory, it is very interesting that in hypnosis components of the personality very similar to subpersonalities of the multiple personality were found also in normal individuals (Watkins and Watkins, 1979-80; Bowers and Brecher, 1955; Watkins, 1993; Lynn et al., 1994; Merskey, 1992; Rickeport, 1992; Barret, 1995). For example, Bowers and Brecher (1955) reported interesting material involved in the emergence of multiple personality structure under hypnosis. The authors conclude that this structure was not produced by the hypnosis, but preceded the beginning of the hypnotic work. The patient in the case under discussion had not shown the multiple structure in clinical and psychological examinations prior to the hypnosis. In his conscious state the patient was not aware of his three underlying personalities, each of which reported distinctive dream material and Rorschach responses.

Conversely, Barret (1995) describes similarities between the states of dreaming and multiple personality disorder including amnesia and other alterations of memory. This suggests the dream character as a hallucinated projection of aspects of the self that can be seen as a prototype for the alter personalities. It corresponds to findings that physiological mechanism for amnesia and the manufacture of alter identities, and related cognitive and personality processes that operate outside conscious awareness occur during dreaming (Barret, 1995). Extreme early trauma may mutate or overdevelop these dissociated parts, inducing them to function in the external world, and thus leading to development of multiple personality disorder. According to these data the dream model parallels the observed phenomena of multiple personality more directly than do explanations relying on waking fantasy processes (Barret, 1995).

6.2. DISSOCIATION AND DREAM FUNCTIONS

Immediate connections between dreams and the dissociated structure of the personality could represent alter personalities that occur on parallel levels - on the one hand in dreams and on the other, in hypnosis. These connections are exhibited in a case study by Salley (1988):

"Frank is a 37-year-old white man with multiple personality. His biological father was incarcerated when he was born. Frank lived with his maternal grandparents soon after his birth. The multiple organization began at the age of 6 years when he was sent to his biological mother's home. His mother had remared an alcoholic who abused Frank physically and emotionally. A history of blackouts, amnesia for certain actions, fugues, abrupt personality changes, and historical conversions has been well documented from medical records dating back to Frank's late teens. His multiple past diagnoses have included chronic undifferentiated schizophrenia (the most common diagnosis), organic brain syndrome, inadequate personality, and seizure disorder. This patient had a long history of appearing on hospital grounds in a state of seizure with no memory for person, situation or past. The memory would typically return within a few days for all but a brief period of time, ranging from a few days to month just preceding the seizure. His life since his late teens has been an almost constant pattern of hospitalizations and fugues that have taken him all over the country.

Early in treatment, before the existence of the multiple personality organization was known a tentative diagnosis of psychogenic fugue was entertained. Hypnotherapy was used to attempt to uncover lost memory. An ISH (Internal Self Helper) was discovered through hypnosis who identified himself as Self, a protector of Frank. Self in somnambulistic trance, explained that the seizures resulted from a struggle between Frank and Self at those times when Frank would resist regaining consciousness after a blackout and Self would to attempt to force him to be conscious. Self stated that his only line of communication with Frank was through dreams and that he would create a dream that would explain to Frank the functions of the seizures. Out of trance, Frank as was typical, had no memory of what had occurred in hypnosis. That night Frank dreamt that he was standing on a pedestal and two voices were shouting at him; one voice shouting "Yes!" and the other "No!" The vibrations from the shouting were so intense that the pedestal began to shake and split open, whereupon he fell to the ground shaking. Free association to the elements of the dream led Frank to relate the shaking to his seizures and the screaming to internal conflict and his resistance to regaining consciousness after a blackout. In the two years since he had this dream, he has experienced no recurrence of the hysterical seizures. In this dream sequence, a dissociated aspect of personality organization predicted and apparently created a dream to communicate with another aspect of the personality."

Frank had 13 personalities, two of which claimed a dream production function. These personalities were able to organize and create dreams for the communication with the host personality.

Further literature also shows the clinical evidence that "dream work" of the ego is operative in both the representation of a separate self in dreams and in alter personalities (Brenner, 1996, 1999, 2001). For example, a striking relationship of dreams and dissociative states was demonstrated in a patient with multiple personality disorder, who, in her usual state of consciousness reported a very distressing dream: she was watching a young girl being sexually abused by an unknown man while an unknown woman was holding her down. A number of days later, a young girl alter spontaneously emerged in a session, who described an eerily first-hand experience. This alter had no awareness that the dream had been reported and the patient had amnesia for the time when her alter was "out" giving her report of the trauma (Brenner, 1996).

Similarly, Barrett (1994, 1996) reported cases of multiple personality with alters appearing as dream characters, or alters who could orchestrate dream content, and even cases of integration occurring within a dream. He discussed the strong potential of these dream characteristics to facilitate the therapy of dissociative disorders.

However, in contrast to Saley's case, Epstein (1964) reported cases when recurrent dreams occur episodically during sleep or waking, and also as a seizure content in temporal lobe epileptics. As is known, such recurrent dreams occur also in individuals who are clinically nonepileptics and may arise after a traumatic event.

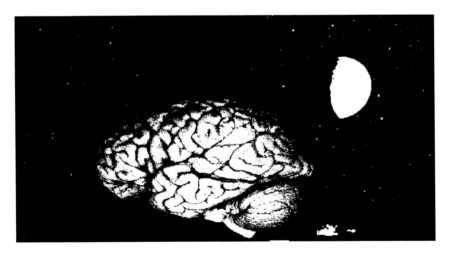

Figure 13. Dreaming brain.

6.3. DREAM AS REFLECTION OF DISSOCIATIVE PROCESSES

Alter personalities with dreaming functions thus support the view of the dream as a reflection of the self-monitoring dissociated system in the study of Gabel (1989), who shows important connections and similarities between hypnotic states and dreams. From these connections among complex theory and dream production in multiple personality we may support the view that the dreams of a healthy person also represent a reflection of interactions and an arrangement of dissociated components of the personality. The relationship of hypnotic and dream processes, in the case of alters with dream functions shows a closer connection between hypnosis and dreams. Conversely, in their manifestations, the consequences of posthypnotic suggestion are very similar to some psychopathological phenomena (Huston, Skehow, and Ericson, 1934) that are induced by the mechanism of repression and lead to a dissociated state by lowering the corresponding psychic content under the limit of consciousness. Probably both repression and posthypnotic suggestion are connected to subliminal perception and information processing. In this context Stross and Shevrin (1962, 1968, 1969) suggest that alterations of the thought contents under hypnosis can be observed during investigations of "freely evoked images" after the subliminal presentation. Their major conclusion was that hypnosis leads to heightened access to subliminal stimuli. As a result, Stross and Shevrin concluded that thought organization during hypnosis shares some common elements with thought organization during dreaming. Other studies (Silverstein, 1993; Fischer, 1954; Poetzl, 1960), supporting their conclusion, showed that subliminally presented images were found in dreams.

All the same, Salley's findings (Salley, 1988) and other documented dream works with patients suffering from multiple personality disorder (Putnam, 1989; Jeans, 1976; Marmer, 1980a,b), where dreams can play an important role in uncovering buried trauma or identifying secretive alters, represent important data for research and the resolution of the problem concerning the relationship between dream and hypnosis. It suggests that individual alter personalities may shape or create dreams separately from other alters. In addition, these data support Gabel's hypothesis that dream material in healthy persons being similar to that of multiple personalities or to the similar phenomenon observed in patients with traumatic neurosis (Ferenczi, 1934; Levitan, 1980), demonstrates the personality system of dissociated and disowned experiences.

A comparable paradigm for dreams establishes connection of recurrent dreams and nightmares after trauma (Hartmann, 1998). A traumatized person may dream first about the actual trauma, but not always. Later, the dreams appear to deal with dominant emotion and about original sensory input from the actual trauma. The dreams contextualize, i.e. they find a picture context for the emotional concern represented by a dominant emotion. This contextualization can be seen in stressful situations, in pregnancy, or in patients whose lives are dominated by one emotion. This pattern may be paradigmatic for all dreams but often it is difficult to detect it in ordinary dreams, because there may be a number of other relatively smaller emotional concerns that interact with dominant one (Hartmann, 1998). The contextualization found in traumatized patients corresponds to transformation of unconscious contents into the dream symbols according to Jung (1972c) or Silberer who called it a "functional phenomenon" that transforms thoughts into images and changes the unconscious thoughts into the dream contents (Silberer, 1909; Silber, 1970).

Similarly there are findings that show empirical foundation for a self psychology of dreaming (Fiss, 1986). Laboratory evidence demonstrated that dreaming serves three primary functions: 1) the maintenance of self-cohesiveness, 2) the restoration of a crumbling or fragmenting self, and 3) the development of new psychic structures. This supports Kohut's view of the dream as perfect (metaphorical) description of the entire patients "self" the so-called "self state dream." Similarly also further studies support the view that dreams provide access to underlying personality structure, as well as its defensive and adaptive structures (Guralnik, Levin, and Schmeidler, 1999).

In the neural network models, dreaming represents the hyperconnective process in the autoassociative net with rapid information processing corresponding to neurobiological findings that during REM sleep new synaptic connections are being created (Hartmann, 1998; Bob, 2004).

The above leads us to propose the hypothesis for future research that the dreams of healthy persons also represent a reflection of interactions and order of dissociated components of the personality. In this context a dream discontinuity is similar to discontinuity of consciousness in waking state that is connected to dissociation in the presence of marked changes in memory, identity or consciousness. Extreme intensity of discontinuous jumps in the dream occur in pathological cases such as recurrent dreams, nightmares after trauma (Hartman, 1998) and also in patients with traumatic neurosis (Ferenczi, 1934; Levitan, 1980; Bob, 2004) which documents that in the dreams emerge dissociated and disowned experiences. Immediate connections between dreams and the dissociated structure of the personality represent alter personalities in multiple personality disorder that occur on parallel levels - on the one hand in dreams and on the other, in hypnosis or in personality alterations of the subject. These connections are exhibited in reported case studies and documented dream works with patients suffering from multiple personality disorder (Putnam, 1989; Saley, 1988; Jeans, 1976; Marmer, 1980a,b; Bob, 2004a), where dreams can play an important role in uncovering buried trauma or identifying secretive alters. This suggests that individual alter personalities may shape or create dreams separately from other alters.

Further literature also shows the clinical evidence that "dream work" of the ego is operative in both the representation of a separate self in dreams and in alter personalities (Brenner, 1996, 1999, 2001). For example, a striking relationship of dreams and dissociative states was demonstrated in a patient with multiple personality disorder, who, in her usual state of consciousness reported a very distressing dream: she was watching a young girl being sexually abused by an unknown man while an unknown woman was holding her down. A number of days later, a young girl alter spontaneously emerged in a session, who described an eerily first-hand experience. This alter had no awareness that the dream had been reported and the patient had amnesia for the time when her alter was "out" giving her report of the trauma (Brenner, 1996, 1999, 2001).

Similarly, Barrett (1994, 1996) reported cases of multiple personality with alters appearing as dream characters, or alters who could orchestrate dream content, and even cases of integration occurring within a dream. Barret (1994, 1995, 1996) discussed the strong potential of these dream characteristics to facilitate the therapy of dissociative disorders in the context of similarities between the states of dreaming and multiple personality disorder including amnesia and other alterations of memory. This suggests the dream character as a hallucinated projection of aspects of the self that can be seen as a prototype for the alter personalities. It corresponds to findings that physiological mechanism for amnesia and the manufacture of alter identities, and the cognitive and personality processes that operate outside conscious awareness occur during dreaming. Extreme early trauma may mutate or overdevelop these dissociated parts, inducing them to function in the external world, and thus leading to development of multiple personality disorder. According to these data the dream model parallels the observed phenomena of multiple personality more directly than do explanations relying on waking fantasy processes. These data correspond to findings that in hypnosis components of the personality very similar to subpersonalities of the multiple personality were found also in normal individuals (Watkins and Watkins, 1979-80; Bowers and Brecher, 1995; Watkins, 1993; Lynn et al., 1994; Merskey, 1992; Rickeport, 1992; Barret, 1995).

These findings suggest that dissociated discrete behavioural states are projected into the dream scenery during the dreaming process in REM sleep when new synaptic connections and new activity patterns are created. It corresponds to findings which suggest that dreams may be understood as reflection of self-monitoring dissociated system (Gabel, 1989) that compensate emotional tension and influence learning process and memory (Rotenberg, 1992).

6.4. DREAMING, SWITCHING OF NEURAL PATTERNS AND DISSOCIATIVE STATES

A characteristic feature of dreaming is discontinuous switching of neuronal activation patterns which is a result of phasic bursts of acetylcholine that activates otherwise quiescent neurons (Kahn and Hobson, 1993; Faw, 1997; Kahn et al., 1997, 2000, 2002; Stickgold et al., 2001; Hobson and Pace-Schot, 2002; Bob, 2006). According to the theory of Mamelak and Hobson this switching in neuronal firing patterns has its cognitive correlate in the discontinuous jumps between dream events due to activity of cholinergic pontogeniculoocipital (PGO) system (Kahn and Hobson, 1993; Kahn et al., 1997, 2000, 2002). Disinhibition in the forebrain structures produces not only neural network errors but is driven far from equilibrium. The strong phasic cholinergic input, in the form of pontogeniculoocipital bursts is likely linked to self-organization and chaotic processes and these self-organized processes induced due to activity of pontogeniculoocipital system were on cognitive level identified with dream images (Kahn and Hobson, 1993; Kahn et al., 1997). During dreaming continuous processes occur that run during long segments of the dream. These processes are sometimes disturbed by incoherences and significant changes in the dream scenery (Kahn and Hobson, 1993; Stickgold, et al. 1994). Decreased inhibitory activity in the noradrenergic locus coeruleus and the serotonergic dorsal raphe nucleus leads to increased excitability of REM-on cells that occur in several brain stem nuclei. Among the disinhibited systems are also neurons of the pontine reticular formation. Particularly interesting group of REM-on cells are the so-called "PGO burst" cells in the cholinergic pedunculopontine nucleus (CH6). These pontine formation neurons fire single spikes during waking when they are assumed to enhance sensorimotor integration (Callaway et al., 1987) but discharge in clusters during the REM sleep (Hobson, 1990; Hobson and McCarley, 1977; Kahn et al., 2000; Kahn and Hobson, 1993; Quattrochi et al., 1989; Stickgold et al., 2002). On the other hand there is evidence that pontogeniculoocipital (PGO) activity is correlated with increased firing in the visual cortex and in the lateral geniculate bodies and it probably leads to more dream images when is reached the threshold frequency in neuronal networks of the visual cortex that is necessary for image formation (Callaway et al., 1987; Kahn and Hobson, 1993; Singer, 1989b; Stickgold et al., 2002).

There is also strong evidence that complex motor patterns are governed at the level of the brain stem but blocked at the level of the spinal cord. Since the PGO-related neuronal firing encodes some aspects of these motor commands, it is possible that the forebrain incorporates information about this fictive movement into the dream (Kahn and Hobson, 1993; Porte and Hobson, 1996).

In the dreams the so-called dream bizarreness occurs that represents unlike elements in the dream such as discontinuities of time, place, person, object and action as well as incongruities of these same features. Discontinuities include abrupt shifts in dream narrative, interruptions in orientational stability and inappropriate matching of different characters, objects or scenes of the dream. According to self-organization theory qualitative changes in cognition will occur in REM sleep due to the incorporation of bottom-up images whose intensity and frequency are assumed to increase during REM sleep. These images are generated when neural processes self-organize as a result of increased cholinergic and decreased aminergic input onto forebrain structures (Kahn and Hobson, 1993). Relationship between bursts of PGO activity and dream mentation (Stickgold, et al., 1994) suggests that non-continuous jumps in neuronal processes correspond to qualitative shifts in dream segments that are linked to discontinuities. Similarly the state-dependent neural network model leads to the understanding of dreaming as a self-organizing process and predict that new sequences of neuronal events may emerge due to a burst of PGO activity (Kahn and Hobson, 1993; Stickgold et al., 2002). Under these conditions the brain becomes sensitive to small disturbances in the neuronal firing pattern of some brain cells and may amplify such disturbances causing a bifurcation from its reference state. It leads to situation when in which many neurons are recruited into a homogeneous oscillation of increasing frequency and amplitude and the result is a traveling wave and an epileptic seizure (Kaczmarek and Babloyantz, 1977; Kahn and Hobson, 1993). This example is particularly important because there are many similarities between the REM sleep, PGO wave and the epileptic spike and wave complex (Elazar and Hobson, 1985; Kahn and Hobson, 1993). Cognitively these bursts may lead to dream bizarreness when the PGO waves induce neuronal patterns which are incongruous with patterns of actually running dream or on the other hand when the PGO waves may act as environmental fluctuations that destabilize the existing neuronal organization with following chaotic state and self-organization of a new neuronal pattern linked to new cognitive correlate that lead to dream discontinuity (Kahn and Hobson, 1993). When the occurrence of dreaming with PGO bursts is modeled as dichotomous Markov noise a rich set of transitions is observed that more accurately reflects the dreaming state. In these multiple transitions instead of a relative continuity in dream narrative, different images compete for expression with the resulting dream discontinuities (Kahn and Hobson, 1993). This competition and interference of dream images (Rotenberg, 1992; Tender and Kramer, 1971) are connected to conjunction errors between mismatching attributes of dream images (Kahn et al., 1997) that similarly as in waking states may be understood as a manifestation of dissociative states corresponding to competition of dissociated contents that in cases of strong competition may lead to non-linear chaotic transitions (Bob, 2003b; Bob, 2006).

Psychological dissociation and chaotic processes in the brain provide links that suggest significant connections between processes in the human mind and brain physiology. Dissociation on the neurophysiological level understood in the connection to chaotic competition offers interesting framework for understanding connections between probable neural correlate of dissociated states that could represent burst of epileptiform activity and psychophysiological processes during dreaming. Several evidence in the literature also referred that dreams are connected to dissociation and may serve as reflection of dissociated state (Gabel, 1989; Bob, 2004; Bob, 2006). These connections enhance understanding of dreams as dissociative states and support the concept of dissociation understood in the connection to chaos and epileptiform activity. This suggests an integrative approach to relationship between mind and brain, and refers to depth psychological dimensions of dreams that can serve as a unique instrument for therapy and understanding of the human mind.

Chapter 7

BRAIN AND CONSCIOUSNESS

7.1. CONSCIOUSNESS AND THE BINDING PROBLEM

In a classical paper on visual consciousness Crick and Koch (1992) express the view that the main problem of visual consciousness may not be resolved only as a simple consequence of synhronization among large groups of neurons. They suggest that a new scientific framework for the study of consciousness comparable to the formulation of the quantum mechanics in physics may be needed. As a reason for that opinion they emphasize the so-called "binding problem", which means that a seen object in the brain is represented by the groups of synchronized excited neurons that are located at different parts of the brain. According to recent findings different parts of visual information are processed in different parts of the brain but it is not known whether spatial convergency is needed for the synthesis of processed information. The hypothetical center for information convergency was termed "Cartesian theatre." Recent neuroscience, however, has not located a distinct place in which distributed information in the brain comes together. Additionally, there is evidence that neocortical processing is distributed during all sensory and motor functions (Singer, 1993, 2001).

The predominant view in neuroscience of consciousness is that neuronal synchronization is a phenomenon that is necessary for the large scale integration of distributed neuronal activities. There is increasing experimental evidence that coherent neuronal assemblies in the brain are functionally linked by phase synchronization among simultaneously recorded EEG signals and that this time-dependent synchrony between various discrete neuronal assemblies represents neural substrate for mental representations such as perception, cognitive functions and memory (Lachaux, Rodriguez, Martinerie and Varela, 1999; Varela, Lachaux, Rodriguez, and Martinerie, 2001; Rees et al., 2002; Summerfield et al., 2002). These functions are related to distributed macroscopic patterns of neuronal activity which involve multiple neuronal subsystems bound into a coherent whole (Braitenberg, 1978; van Putten and Stam, 2001). According to recent data, a mechanism that enables binding of distributed macroscopic patterns of neuronal activity, represented by neural assemblies, into the coherent whole is still unresolved and represents a fundamental problem in neuroscience (i.e., binding problem; how the brain codes and integrates distributed neural activities during processes connected to perception, cognition and memory) (Arp, 2005; Fidelman, 2005; Lee, Williams, Breakspear, and Gordon, 2003; Woolf and Hameroff, 2001).

The theory of feature binding originates in concept of distributed coding and states that neurons involved in the processing of a single object will tend to synchronize their firing, while simultaneously desynchronizing their firing from the remaining neurons not involved in the processing of the object (von der Malsburg and Schneider, 1986). An essential feature of neuronal assembly coding is that individual neurons or subsystems can participate at different times in an almost unlimited number of different assemblies (Sannita, 2000; Varela et al., 2001). The same neurons can participate in different perceptual events and different combinations of these neurons can represent different perceptual objects. Synchronization of these different perceptual objects is related to the integration of perceptions into a coherent whole (Singer and Gray, 1995). A candidate mechanism for the integration or binding of distributed brain activities is the so-called gamma activity, i.e. high frequency oscillations of 40 Hz, but often varying from 30 to 90 Hz. This activity occurs synchronously across brain regions and underlies the integration of diverse brain activities (Singer and Gray, 1995). Although the majority of research on feature binding has focused on synchronous gamma activity (35-50 Hz), there is evidence that synchronous activities in other frequency bands may also participate in functional integration of distributed neural activities into the coherent whole (Bressler, Coppola, and Nakamura, 1993; Lee et al., 2003).

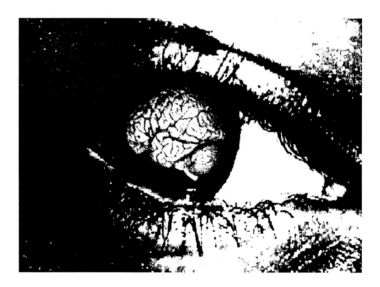

Figure 14. Self-reflective brain.

A solution of the binding problem may lay within the fundamental problem of consciousness in modern neuroscience. Predominant opinion is that consciousness emerges from a dynamical nucleus of persisting reverberation and interactions of neural groups (John, 2002). For example, Tononi and Edelman (2000) emphasize that consciousness is re-entry of neural signals via changes of complexity and entropy in the central nervous system. Libet (1998) suggests that subjective experience represents a field emerging from neural synchronization and coherence, and is not reducible to any physical process (see also John, 2002). In accordance with Libet, Squires (1998) maintains that consciousness may be understood as a primitive component of the world including specific qualities of subjective experience (qualia) that can not be reduced to any other physical quality (John, 2002).

7.2. NEUROPHYSICS OF CONSCIOUSNESS

Regarding the binding problem Marshall (1989) suggests a non-conventional concept for the binding of distributed information and hypothesizes that there exists neither classical physical structure nor neurophysiological substrate suitable for explaining consciousness. Marshall focuses his attention on the "quantum wholeness" of initially interacting but (in the future) spatially distributed subsystems. Main of his suggestions regarding quantum physical substrate of consciousness was that in the quantum reality the non-local instant correlations between spatially distributed parts of the system are possible, independently of any connecting signal between them that could explain unity of consciousness during distributed information processing. Beck and Eccles (1992) suggest a similar theoretical proposal of neurotransmiter release from the presynaptic part of the neuron into the synaptic cleft that has probability less than one. They interpreted this probability as a consequence of the quantum "tunneling effect" that enables a particle to overcome an energetic barrier, which is higher than the energy of the particle (i.e., a phenomenon that is impossible to observe in our macroscopic world described by classical mechanics).

According to Freeman's non-conventional concept (1991, 2000, 2001) the image of the world emerges as a consequence of creating order from non-linear chaotic activity of the large groups of neurons. These nonlinear chaotic processes represent a consequence of high system complexity, when the system involves a large number of complex interlinked and simultaneously active neural assemblies and runs in desynchronized parallel distributed mode which can lead to self-organization (Freeman 1991, 2000, 2001) and typical dynamical instabilities in mental phenomena (Atmanspacher and Fach, 2005).

A new conceptual view provides the so-called "neurogeometry": e.g., a geometrical model of the functional architecture of the primary visual cortex and its pinwheel structure (Petitot, 2003). The problem is to understand how the internal geometry of the visual cortex can produce the geometry of the external space (Petitot, 2003). Solution of the binding problem could principally be explained by similar mathematical approach that is used in the general theory of relativity. According to the theory, distance between two points measured by an observer is influenced by physical state of the observed system. For example, when the observed system significantly changes its velocity that almost reaches the speed of light, the observer registers the distance contraction and increased mass and energy. This effect of movement with significant acceleration leading to accumulation of high mass and energy is according to general theory of relativity likely equivalent to influence of gravitational field. For example, high mass and energy accumulated in the black hole likely cause similar effects of distance contraction. This may implicate that distance between two points in the brain must not be the same from the point of view of external observer in comparison to internal observer, which is subject's mind itself. These effects are mathematically interpreted as changes of space metrics caused by physical processes. Because even the time significantly changes during these processes, relativity theory therefore provides heuristic possibility to use the space-time geometry as a universal description for macrocosm, microcosm and possibly for the human mind by language of mathematics, similarly as Plato thought (Bob, 2008b).

The ideas outlined were considerably developed by Roger Penrose in his books and scientific papers that represent well-known contribution to the quantum theory of human consciousness (Penrose, 1989, 1994, 2001; Hameroff and Penrose, 1995, 1996; Penrose and Hameroff, 1996; Woolf and Hameroff, 2001; Hagan, Hameroff, and Tuszynski, 2002). The starting point of Penrose's analysis represents cosmology and the requirement to formulate a quantum theory of gravity that is important for unifying quantum mechanics with Einstein's general theory of relativity. The crucial problem at this point is the process of measurement during microphysical processes in quantum mechanics. In a classical solution by Bohr (called the Copenhagen interpretation) a collection of possibilities (e.g., all possible trajectories connecting two spatially distributed points) in the development of the system (characterized by wave function Ψ) is reduced to one macroscopic actualized possibility (e.g., one of the set of possible trajectories) by measurement or observation performed on the quantum system (Laurikainen 1988; Penrose 1994; Wheeler and Zurek, 1983). This process emerges in the transition from the quantum reality of possibilities (world of microphysics), characterized by the wave function Ψ, to the macroscopic world of things, characterized by its "sharpness" in the space and time. Penrose (1994) called this process subjective reduction of quantum possibilities. This classical concept of reduction of the wave function led to the well-known Schrödinger's cat paradox. The paradox demonstrates the conflict between quantum theory and macroscopic observations performed on the quantum mechanical system. In a thought experiment, a living cat is placed into a box along with a bottle containing a poison. There is, in the bottle, a very small amount of a radioactive material. If even a single atom of the radioactive material decays during the experiment, a relay mechanism with radioactive detector will trip a hammer, which will, in turn, break the bottle with poison and kills the cat. The observer cannot know whether or not an atom of the substance has decayed and the cat is killed. According to the Copenhagen interpretation, the cat is in a superposition of states and is both dead and alive (Penrose, 1994, 2004; Wheeler and Zurek, 1983). When the observer opens the box, the superposition is lost by the interaction with the observer and the cat becomes dead or alive. According to Penrose, a solution of this problem can be found in the theory of quantum gravity that might explain spontaneous reduction of the superposition i.e., objective reduction independently of measurement or observation (Penrose, 1994, 2001, 2002). That mathematical formulation of Penrose's ideas is linked to the theory of Newtonian quantum gravity that represents quantization of gravity in the Newtonian space and time (Ghirardi, Grassi, and Pearle, 1990). Objective reduction according to Penrose is linked to non-computability which corresponds to an interpretation of Gödel's theorem. The theorem postulates that it is not possible to express the whole world by any system of mathematical axioms (Penrose, 1994). From the philosophical point of view objective reduction can be interpreted as a non-predictable spontaneous expression of a Platonic idea (or archetype) into the world of things; at this point Penrose's opinion is similar to Jung's or Pauli's view of archetypes as transcendental reality (Pauli called Ψ the Platonic world) that constitutes empirical reality (Laurikainen 1988).

Penrose (1997, p. 1) wrote: "Since I shall be talking about the physical world in terms of physical theories which underlie its behaviour, I shall also have to say something about another world, the Platonic world of absolutes, in its particular role as the world of mathematical truth … as a structure precisely governed according to ('timeless') world of mathematics..." This problem, although formulated in modern language, leads to dilemma, whether mathematical truth is only an idealization of the external world or represents a realistic entity. This is an old problem known from the Plato's time, usually formulated as a conflict between realism and nominalism in medieval philosophical history (i.e. the nominalism, in contrast to realism, emphasizes that abstract terms, general terms, or universals do not represent objective real existents, but are merely names). The problem of modern mathematics emerges in the dilemma as to whether or not mathematics is only a language of description of the world, or whether it is a law of the world. The remarkable ability of mathematics to describe the world may lead to the opinion that the physical world emerges from the Platonic world of mathematics. In a similar way Penrose dealt with the role of the objective reduction in brain functions that enable to create an inner psychological world, in a similar way as the external world of things is created. Penrose links this objective reduction process with quantum gravity. Because the quantum-gravity state may enable the so-called quantum entanglement of distributed neurons the approach may resolve the binding problem of distributed and synchronized neural populations (Crick, 1994; Crick and Clark, 1994; Penrose, 1994, 2001; Woolf and Hameroff, 2001). Penrose has utilized in a way similar to Marshall (1989) the model of biological coherent quantum states which was initially proposed by Fröhlich (1968, 1970, 1975). These coherent quantum states, according to the hypothesis, are caused by electron conformational dynamics of proteins of the neural cytoskeleton (Penrose 1994) and are linked to inter- and intra-cellular communication in the central nervous system (Zaccai, Massoulié, and David, 1998). Distributed information in the brain, according to this view, could be "non-locally" linked by electron conformational dynamics of microtubule structures (Penrose, 1994, 1997). The principle of non-locality is analogical to Jung's principle of synchronicity as an acausal connecting principle that describes the temporally coincident occurrences of acausal events (Mansfield and Spiegelman, 1989, 1991). This principle of acausal connections was linked by Jung to his concept of archetypes and the collective unconscious, which represent a governing dynamics (analogous to chaotic self-organization) that underlie the whole human experience fragmented into divided states of consciousness (Bob, 2003b, 2004, 2008b).

Application of these heuristic hypotheses to brain research implicates that brain metrics from the point of view of external observer, who sees the brain as an object, must not be the same as the "metrics" of the brain's interpreter that enables the subject's consciousness. From this point of view the binding problem may be resolved by non-existent distance among the parts of the brain from the point of view of brain's interpreter, because of different space metrics that enables brain synchronization and coherence (Bob, 2008b). Analogical situation may occur in the so-called quantum non-locality. The non-locality in principle means entanglement between two initially interacting micro-objects across the distance with zero lag correlation. At this point both relativity theory and quantum theory, or their prospective synthesis in quantum theory of gravity, may be potentially useful for the study of brain and consciousness. Consideration of these heuristic hypotheses significantly opens possible view of brain processes in the context of fundamental physical theories that could play a key role for research of physical aspects of consciousness.

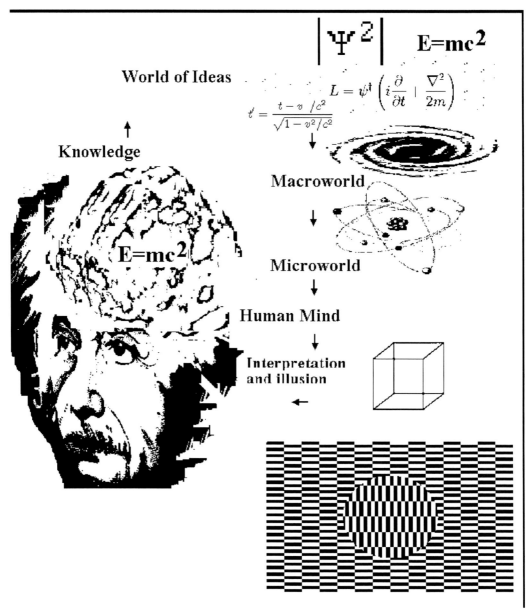

Figure 15. Platonic ideas coming into human mind through the physical world that emerges from the Platonic world of mathematics.

Chapter 8

CHAOS, SELF-ORGANIZATION AND DISSOCIATED MIND

8.1. CHAOS, BRAIN AND COGNITION

The concept of dynamical chaos was for the first time developed by French mathematician Henri Poincaré (1854-1912), who studied predictability in a system behavior and found that chaotic randomness does not mean a true randomness because it is caused by unpredictability and sensitivity with respect to stimuli that influence system behavior and determine disproportional changes. The sensitivity is related to the quality of prediction of a system's behavior regarding an information loss over time that leads to decrease in the accuracy of prediction of later system's development. In his "Science and method" (p. 68) Poincaré wrote: "A very small, unnoticeable cause can determine a visible very large effect; in this case we claim that this effect is a product of random. . . However, even if the natural laws were perfectly known, we will ever be able to know the initial conditions with some approximation. If this allows us to know the future with the same approximation that is all we want. We will say that the phenomenon is foreseeable, that it is governed by laws; however this is not always the case, it is possible that very small initial differences lead to very large one in the final state. . ."

Although this nonlinear mathematical approach to the so-called chaotic phenomena and complexity in nature has its roots in the Poincaré's work in the last years of 19th century, its application to the field of psychology and neuroscience is relatively new. Aim for using this method is the understanding of relatively short periods in the behaviour of a system which are extremely sensitive to very little changes (the so-called sensitivity to initial conditions). This sensitivity during critical times characterizes initiation of new trends in the system's evolution which later emerge as very different macroscopic patterns of neural activity and mental processes (Elbert et al, 1994; Freeman, 1983, 1991, 2000; Birbaumer et al., 1995; Kantz and Schreiber, 1997; Meyer-Lindenberg et al., 2002; van Putten and Stam, 2001; Faure and Korn 2001; Globus and Arpaia 1994; Korn and Faure 2003). Chaotic transitions probably emerge in a wide variety of cognitive phenomena and possibly may be linked to specific changes during development of mental disorders such as depression or schizophrenia (Korn and Faure, 2003; Melancon and Joanette, 2000; Gottschalk et al., 1995; Barton, 1994; Huber et al., 1999; Paulus and Braff, 2003) and might underlie psychological hypersensitivity to outside stimuli and their pathological processing. A possible role of chaotic transitions in dissociative states and disorders is at this time unknown. There are several hypotheses that link the dissociation to critical chaotic shifts of discrete behavioural states (Putnam, 1997) and underlying competitive neural assemblies which form mental representations of dissociated states (Bob 2003b) with the resulting self-organization of behavioural patterns during critical periods (Pediaditakis, 1992; Sel, 1997). Because of chaotic nature of epileptiform discharges (Velazquez et al., 2003), there is evidence suggesting possible importance of chaotic transitions in dissociative states and disorders. The evidence is based on relatively frequent occurrence of epileptic discharges or epileptiform abnormalities documented in dissociated patients who are victims of child abuse (Coons et al., 1989; Teicher et al., 1993, 2003; Ito et al., 1993) during dissociative states such as depersonalization (Sierra and Berrios, 1998), multiple personality disorder (Mesulam, 1981; Benson, Miller and Signer 1986; Spiegel, 1991; Bob, 2003b, 2007a), dissociative disorders not otherwise specified and dissociative seizures (the so-called pseudoepilepsy) (Bowman and Coons, 2000) and on the other hand there is evidence of relatively frequent ictal as well as interictal dissociative symptoms in epileptics including multiple personality disorder (Schenk and Bear, 1981; Hersch et al., 2002; Ahern et al., 1993). There is also recent discussion regarding an influence of childhood trauma on kindling in temporolimbic structures and resulting epileptiform pathology of patients with dissociative disorders (Post et al., 1995; Putnam, 1997; Teicher et al., 2003). With respect to the evidence of chaotic nature of epileptic discharges (Faure and Korn, 2001; Korn and Faure, 2003; Elbert et al., 1994; Freeman, 1991; Lehnertz, 1999; Velazquez et al., 2003) this suggests the hypothesis of possible chaotic process mainly in temporolimbic structures which might underlie dynamics of dissociative states and development of dissociative disorders.

There is also relevant assumption that chaotic neural mechanism is related to concomitant chaotic psychological process (Pediaditakis, 1992; Sel, 1997; Putnam, 1997; Bob, 2003b, 2007a; Bob et al., 2008). Dissociation on the psychological level is closely related to confusion and situation such as "I do not know what to do", when any possible solution is not sufficient. This lead to competition among very high number of prototype mental images representing a possible solution. These mental representations of possible solutions constitute different behavioural patterns and strategies including identity (who I am in a certain situation and behaviour). On neural level this state is probably linked to a large number of complex and interlinked neural states which lead to extreme instability with respect to competition of many patterns of neural activity. In animal models this corresponds to the so-called winnerless competition when any solution in a stressful situation is not found (Korn and Faure, 2003). This winnerless competition has been also suggested as one of important mechanisms which cause the neural chaos (Korn and Faure, 2003). The winnerless competition thus might also serve as a behavioural model of human cognition that leads to dissociated state. Chaotic behaviour as a consequence of winnerless competition may produce extremely different outcomes with respect to previous state because of their sensitivity to initial conditions (the so-called butterfly effect). These extremely different outcomes may emerge by abrupt shifts in mood and behaviour which are typical for dissociative states.

The cases of 'antagonistic' competition or the winnerless competition among neural assemblies leading to chaos therefore does not mean only an absence of order and unpredictability but the term chaos implies the idea of underlying structure and the potential for describing a complex system with the aid of relatively simple mathematical formulations with a basis in nonlinear mathematics. Generally, chaos in the neural system may leads to a low-dimensional aperiodic signal that may be used for describing behavior resulting from very many degrees of freedom in systems with very high complexity (Elbert et al. 1994; Tirsch et al. 2004). Freeman proposed that brain chaos probably arises from the competition of two or more parts of the brain represented by neuronal assemblies (Freeman, 1991; Elbert et al. 1994) and this process may represents neurophysiological substrate for competition of mental representations (Bob, 2003b).

8.2. CHAOS AND EPILEPTIFORM PROCESS

Chaos leads to an often instantaneous reduction of excitatory thresholds of many neural populations not excited in that particular combination before (Freeman, 1991; Elbert *et al.* 1994). Additionally, chaos may lead to a process known as bifurcation. Bifurcations characterize networks that are sensitive to very weak changes of initial conditions. As Freeman suggested that the bifurcations may lead neural activity, which can be observed as unexpected original ideas or in pathological cases as epileptic paroxysms (Elbert *et al.* 1994; Freeman, 1991). A characteristic feature of neural activity due to brain chaos is synchronous collective activity - a burst (Freeman 1991). The burst waves often have a frequency of about 40 Hz and high amplitudes. Increasing competition as a consequence of failure of associative connections without possibility to agree on a common frequency of oscillations leads after extremely intense and hypersynchronous gamma rhythms to epileptiform discharges and decreasing gamma oscillations (Medvedev, 2001, 2002; Alarcon et al., 1995; Allen et al., 1992; Fisher et al., 1992; Huang and White, 1989). In this context could be important that epileptiform activity has been suggested as an antibinding mechanism which is related to a failure of associative connections between neural assemblies (Medvedev, 2001, 2002) and corresponding fragmentation of related mental representations characteristic for dissociative states. Chaotic self-organization during these processes leads to pathological states such as epileptic paroxysms (Elger et al., 2000; Korn and Faure, 2003) or other manifestations of epileptiform activity when competitive neural assemblies remain disassociated or as unexpected original ideas due to successful creating of new associations during the chaotic competition (Elbert et al., 1994; Freeman, 1991, 2000, 2001; Skarda and Freeman, 1987; Mölle et al., 1996; Lutzenberger et al., 1992; Bob, 2003b). According to propositions of PDP models the competition among neural assemblies on the psychological level is correlated by competition among mental representations (e.g. ideas, feelings or memories) and competitive neural assemblies with low associative strength represents neural base for dissociated mental states. The burst waves often have a frequency of about 40 Hz and high amplitudes and this process also may produce epileptic (or epileptiform) activity that represents a typical form of chaotic behavior (Freeman 1991; Elbert et al.1994; Korn and Faure, 2003; Tirsch et al. 2004). Freeman (1991) suggested that chaos underlies the ability of the brain to respond flexibly to the outside world and to generate novel activity patterns, including those that are experienced as fresh ideas. Chaos from this point of view expresses the underlying unpredictable order of attractors and enables the complex behavior of the brain (Freeman 1991, 2000, 2001; Skarda and Freeman 1987).

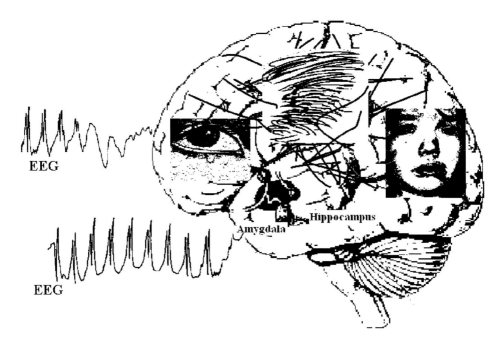

Figure 16. Chaos in the brain and in the mind leading to dissociation could be related to epileptiform activity that presents typical form of chaotic neural organization.

8.3. CHAOS, COGNITIVE CONFLICT AND DISSOCIATION

According to these connections dissociative states understood as competitive states of disintegrated mental representations with resulting chaotic states might explain the mechanism that produces hypersynchronized epileptic activity as a consequence of chaotic competition among neural assemblies and corresponding mental representations of conflicting mental states (Bob, 2003a). In these cases conflict of mental representations may include also interhemispheric competition and dissociation of cerebral hemispheres. On the "macro"-neurophysiological level dissociative processes may be understood in the connection of possible reversible blocking of the transmission from one hemisphere to the other across the corpus callosum and other commissural fibers. It may lead to the competition and chaotic states. This postulate may motivate similarities between some cases of psychic dissociation (or repression) and split brain patients (Galin, 1974) or epilepsy due to defective hemispheric interaction as Ahler et al. (1993) suggested. Dissociation from this point of view may be understood as a blocking of communication between verbal (conscious) left and the other side of the brain (Galin, 1974; Spitzer et al. 2004). On the other hand human creativity represents high level of psychic integration and corresponds to integration of left-hemispheric verbal analytical thought and holistic thought of the right hemisphere (Gallin, 1974; Bogen and Bogen, 1969). These connections suggest direct relationship between Epilepsy/Temporal Lobe Dysfunction model (Putnam 1997) and Cerebral Hemispheric Laterality Model which represents the theory that either an anatomical or a functional disconnection between the two hemispheres of the brain is the source of "double personality" (Putnam, 1989, 1997; Ellenberger, 1970; Quen, 1986). Competitive inter-hemispheric alter personality states connected to dissociated mental representations of corresponding neural assemblies thus suggest the explanation of repeated clinical observations that document laterality differences across alter personalities in multiple personality disorder patients (Brende 1984; Henninger 1992; Le Page et al. 1992; Ahern 1993; Putnam 1997) such as for example in the cases when an intracarotid injection of amobarbital (Wada test) was used to anesthetize the hemisphere and this reproduced the alter personality changes associated with seizure activity in these two patients (Ahern et al. 1993). On the other hand there are controlled test of the laterality that did not find an evidence of shifts in lateralization of galvanic skin response across repeatedly randomized testing of alter-personality states (Putnam 1997) that might be explained by dissociation without inter-hemispheric competition.

8.4. CHAOS AND PANIC ATTACKS

In a study performed in our laboratory (Bob et al., 2006b) we have examined the hypothesis that symptoms of panic disorder also reflect fragmentary, temporally and spatially disorganized memories (Jacobs and Nadel, 1985, 1999; Goodwin, Fergusson, and Horwood, 2005) with resulting chaotic transitions. Evaluation of these phenomena by suitable nonlinear dynamic measures therefore could be useful for assessment of disease evolution and therapeutic progress. Following this proposition we performed the clinical study and examined retrieval of memory associated with anxiety related to a panic attack in 7 patients and retrieval of anxiety related memories in 11 healthy controls along with measurement of EEG (in 8 channels in frontal, central, temporal and parietal regions). Nonlinear data analysis of EEG records suggests a statistically significant increase in degree of chaos measured by largest Lyapunov exponents after retrieval of stressful memory in majority of patients as well as in control subjects. This change was in accordance with intensity of subjective experience during retrieval. The data suggest a role of nonlinear changes of neural dynamics in the processing of stressful memories related to anxiety which might be important for pathophysiology of panic disorder. Because in the brain these nonlinear changes are related to a large number of complex and interlinked neural states which lead to extreme instability with respect to competition of many possible behavioral patterns (Freeman, 2000; Korn and Faure, 2003), the results are consistent with findings that increased chaos probably reflects the competition and interference associated with cognitive conflict (Korn and Faure, 2003; Bob, 2003b). Future perspective of these findings may be a possible explanation of a role of stressful events on epileptiform activity documented in several studies (Teicher et al., 2003, 2006; Post et al., 1995; Putnam, 1997; McNamara and Fogel, 1990; Bystritsky et al., 1999), because epileptiform discharges displays a significantly higher chaotic behavior than normal EEG activity (Velazquez et al., 2003; Stam, 2005). Relationship between traumatic stress and epileptiform discharges thus might be mediated by characteristic nonlinear changes of neural dynamics mainly in the temporal lobe and limbic structures that probably play a major role in the pathophysiology of dissociative disorders, PTSD and other diseases related to childhood abuse.

8.5. CHAOS AND DISSOCIATION DURING HYPNOTIC ABREACTION

In other study performed in our laboratory, hypnotic revivification of dissociated trauma during hypnotic abreaction in two patients has been examined (Bob, 2007a). The clinical experiment for therapeutic and a research purpose was performed along with measurement of bilateral electrodermal activity (EDA) which is modulated mainly by limbic modulation influences and correlates with amygdala activity (Mangina and Beuzeron-Mangina, 1996; Critchley, 2002; Phelps et al., 2001). Recent data also indicate that EDA may be used as a sensitive index of emotion-related sympathetic activity (Dawson, Shell, and Filion, 2000; Critchley, 2002). Nonlinear data analysis of EDA records performed in this study showed a difference between degree of chaos (measured by largest Lyapunov exponents) in hypnotic relaxed state before revivification of the trauma and dissociated state after re-living of the traumatic memory. Results indicate that dissociated state after revivification of the trauma is significantly more chaotic than the state during the hypnotic relaxation before the event. Findings of this study also give a preliminary evidence for a possible role of neural chaos in the processing of the dissociated traumatic memory and suggest an underlying chaotic process in temporolimbic structures related to psychopathology. The chaotic neural process in principle must not be related only to pathological processing but may represent potential existence of a new adaptive level in neurophysiological process, which is actualized for example during successful therapy. Memory reconsolidation that may be related to chaotic neural process probably enables successful transformation from dissociated, automatic and implicitly consolidated traumatic memory mainly in the amygdala, to higher level of conscious experience in the higher-level structures such as medial PFC and hippocampus. This view corresponds to Janet's definition of dissociative state as automatic process which does not fit into current cognitive scheme and without successful reprocessing (and reconsolidation) remains dissociated also during recall of dissociative state because of the specific neural substrate of dissociated memories (Bob, 2007a).

According to the APA definition (American Psychiatric Association 1980, p. 1), "abreaction" represents the release of repressed or suppressed feelings that often follow the traumatic events. According to reported findings in this study is releasing of the traumatic memory related to a chaotic dissociated state. Chaotic state represents extreme sensitivity with respect to very little influences which can significantly affect the future development. This is in accordance with clinical experience that patient during hypnotic abreaction is very sensitive, more suggestible and opened to therapeutic influences and in this moment of great sensitivity, slight comments may enable to create new stable psychological structures, which could be constructive as well as destructive (Bob, 2004c; Bob, 2007).

8.6. Chaos, Limbic Irritability and Dissociation

In nonlinear analysis research programme of our laboratory we also performed the study in which we have examined a relationship between chaotic neural process and cognitive conflict (Bob et al., 2006). This conflict related activation elicits autonomic responses which can be assessed by psychophysiological measures such as heart rate variability calculated as beat to beat R-R intervals (RRI). In our study performed in 30 patients with unipolar depression we have used Stroop word-colour test as an experimental approach to psychophysiological study of cognitive conflict in connection with RRI measurement, psychometric measurement of limbic irritability (LSCL-33) (Teicher et al., 1993), depression (BDI-II) (Beck, 1996) and calculation of largest Lyapunov exponents in nonlinear data analysis of RRI time series. Significant Pearson correlation 0.61 (p<0.01) between largest Lyapunov exponents and LSCL-33 found in this study indicate that a defect of neural inhibition during conflicting Stroop task is closely related to limbic irritability. Because limbic irritability is probably closely related to epileptiform abnormalities in the temporo-limbic structures, this result may point to the neural mechanism connecting trauma related cognitive conflict and epileptiform brain activity. Similar significant correlation 0.58 (p<0.01) we have found also with dissociation measured by dissociative experiences scale (DES). These data suggest that limbic irritability and dissociation are related to neural chaos and may present a pathogenetic mechanism that connect influence of stress and epileptiform discharges, which are also significantly more chaotic in comparison with other brain EEG activities.

Similarly as in the case of cognitive conflict which reflects the competition and interference of many possible behavioral patterns and mental representations during "chaos in the mind", a characteristic feature of neural chaotic states is that they lead to transient periods of high complexity that are coupled to disruption of the temporal structure of integrative brain activity (Dawson, 2004; Fingelkurts et al., 2006; Bob, 2007a; Bob et al., 2006), where the spatio-temporal structure could be either more irregular (uncorrelated randomness with higher complexity) or more regular (excessive order with lower complexity) than normal. Disintegrative processes underlying traumatic stress related memories and dissociative symptoms thus probably reflect fragmentation also on neural level, and are related to specific neural mechanisms that might include chaotic dynamics.

8.7. Chaos and Schizophrenia

Recent data indicate that random-like processes are related to defics in the organization of semantic memory in schizophrenia which is more disorganized and less definable than those of controls with more semantic links and more bizarre and atypical associations and these aspects of schizophrenic cognition are similar to characteristics of chaotic nonlinear dynamical systems (Bob et al., 2007c). In this context it is an open question whether this random-like behavior is realy related to nonlinear dynamics in physiological processes in the schizophrenia brains. The theory of nonlinear dynamical systems and chaos theory on general level deals with deterministic systems that exhibit complex and seemingly random-like behavior. The values of the measured properties of many physiological systems look random and their determinants are often unknown because of high complexity of the factors affecting the phenomena under consideration in physiological research (Elbert et al., 1994; Freeman 2000; Dokoumetzidis et al. 2001; Korn and Faure 2003). Main idea of randomness relies on the concept that every complex system has a large number of degrees of freedom which cannot be directly observed and are manifested through the system's fluctuations (Elbert et al., 1994; Dokoumetzidis et al., 2001; Freeman, 1991, 2000, 2001). Recent research shows that the chaotic deterministic dynamical systems display the random-like behavior often indistinguishable from pure random processes (Elbert et al., 1994; Dokoumetzidis et al., 2001). Although the roots of the chaos theory are in the work of Henry Poincaré (Peterson, 1993), the main results of this interdisciplinary research in the field of physiology are relatively new (Elbert et al., 1994; Freeman, 1991, 2001). In this context the concept of self-organization has been proposed because the chaotic dynamics tends to produce a spontaneous order and patterns of organization in the physiological systems (Elbert et al., 1994; Freeman, 2001; Dokoumetzidis et al., 2001; Korn and Faure, 2003). The self-organization patterns typically are linked to instability states that may enable a new mode of behavior. The sudden phase transitions called bifurcations represents a form of system's behavior which is deterministic and in the state space of the system's behavior is compressed to a subset called the attractor (Elbert et al., 1994; Freeman, 2001; Dokoumetzidis et al., 2001). In the physics state (or phase) space means the abstract multidimensional space in which every possible state of the system corresponds to a unique point in the space that may be visualized by state space diagram. The number of dimensions or parameters of this space represents degree of freedom of the system and every dimension may be represented as axis. For example mechanical system may be described by all possible values of position and momentum or in the thermodynamics states or phases of a chemical system may be described as function of pressure, temperature or composition (Elbert et al. 1994; Dokoumetzidis et al., 2001). Complex macrosystem such as living organism may be therefore described by many state functions such as temperature, blood pressure, electrical activity, for example EEG, ECG, electrodermal activity (EDA) and also other physiological, behavioral or cognitive characteristics (Elbert et al., 1994).

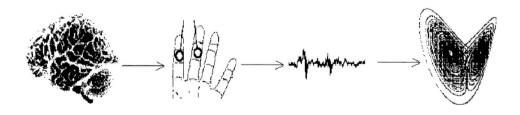

Figure 17. Chaos analysis of electrodermal activity.

Recent findings suggest that methods of chaos theory may represent a useful experimental tool and theoretical model for the study of the complex systems such as the human brain (Korn and Faure, 2003; Melancon and Joanette, 2000; Gottschalk et al., 1995; Huber et al., 1999; Paulus and Braff, 2003; Breakspear, 2006; Bob, 2003b, 2007a; Bob et al., 2006). One of the aims for using this method is understanding of critical sensitive periods (as possible bifurcation points) related to initiation of new trends in the system's evolution that later emerge as very different macroscopic patterns of neural activity and mental processes (Elbert et al., 1994; Freeman, 1991, 2000; Meyer-Lindenberg et al., 2002; Faure and Korn, 2001; Globus and Arpaia, 1994; Korn and Faure, 2003). In the brain the critical sensitive periods are linked to a large number of complex and interlinked neural states which lead to extreme instability with respect to competition of many possible behavioral patterns (Freeman, 2000; Korn and Faure, 2003).

In this context recent data indicate that random-like processes are related to the defect in the organization of semantic memory in schizophrenia which is more disorganized and less definable than those of controls with more semantic links and more bizarre and atypical associations (Davis et al. 1995; Paulsen et al. 1996; Vinogradov et al. 2002). Other studies examined textual analyses of the semantic processing and found that schizophrenic speech is less predictable, more repetitious, and often violates the rules of normal discourse (Manschreck et al., 1979, 1981; Hoffman et al., 1982; Goldberg and Weinberger, 2000). These findings and clinical experience indicate seemingly random patterns in the disorganized cognition in schizophrenia although it is characterized by a complex lawfully mediated behavior (Leroy et al., 2005). These processes are probably closely related to information overload caused by defective attentional filtering and frontal lobe executive dysfunction (Hotchkiss and Harvey, 1990; McGrath, 1991; Goldberg and Weinberger, 2000). Hypothetically it may be explained as random-like chaotic behavior in the neural systems. This pathological information processing might lead to a failure to inhibit activities of irrelevant neural assemblies (Vaitl et al., 2002; Olypher et al., 2006) and pathologically increased neural complexity characterized by an amount of independently active neural assemblies. The explanation is in accordance with findings that chaotic states in deterministic structure of the system occur when the neural process involves a large number of complex interlinked and simultaneously active states which lead to self-organization and high complexity (Korn and Faure, 2003). It is also in accordance with recent data which suggest that chaotic processes likely emerge in a wide variety of cognitive phenomena and might be linked to pathophysiological changes in schizophrenia and other mental disorders (Korn and Faure, 2003; Melancon and Joanette, 2000; Gottschalk et al., 1995; Huber et al., 1999; Paulus and Braff, 2003; Breakspear 2006; Bob, 2003b, 2007a; Bob et al. 2006). From this point of view, pathophysiology of schizophrenia may be related to underlying chaotic neural process mainly in the frontotemporal and limbic structures, which might determine dynamics of schizophrenia and development of the disease (Paulus and Braff, 2003; Breakspear, 2006). One of the sensitive measures of specific pathophysiological changes during pathogenesis of schizophrenia is electrodermal activity (EDA) (Dawson and Schell, 2002; Williams et al., 2002; Schell et al., 2005; Zahn and Pickar, 2005; Bob et al., 2007). These findings strongly suggest that EDA may help to predict treatment outcome and that specific electrodermal dysfunctions may carry prognostic information regarding subsequent symptoms, as well as social and occupational outcome in medicated patients (Dawson and Schell, 2002). For example, the typical results of these studies are that heightened EDA typical for schizophrenia also in medicated patients was significantly correlated with poor short-term symptomatic recovery and that heightened EDA was associated with more disorganized symptoms which suggest that specific patterns of mental and semantic disorganization could be reflected in EDA records (Zahn et al., 1991, 1997; Dawson and Schell, 2002; Schell et al., 2005). These results strongly suggest that when arousal increases beyond the level needed to initiate attention and problem solving it leads to interference in cognitive processing and impaired ability to discriminate between relevant and irrelevant information that cause mental disorganization (Dawson and Schell, 2002; Schell et al., 2005). Recent evidence indicates that EDA is governed by limbic modulation influences and correlates with amygdala activity, but also other structures such as ventromedial and dorsolateral prefrontal cortices, anterior cingulate gyrus, parietal lobe, insula and hippocampus in EDA modulation are involved (Mangina and Beuzeron-Mangina, 1996; Critchley, 2002; Phelps et al., 2001). Typical for EDA is that it reflects activity within the sympathetic axis of the autonomic nervous system and serves as a sensitive index of sympathetic activity (Dawson et al., 2000; Critchley, 2002). Nonlinear measures calculated from EDA thus may serve as characteristics that can be used as an indicator of possible chaotic process in neural systems in comparison of schizophrenic patients with normal control group. This hypothesis is in agreement with our reported study in 40 schizophrenic patients and 40 healthy subjects who were investigated using measurement of bilateral electrodermal activity during rest conditions (Bob et al., 2007c). Results of nonlinear and statistical analysis indicated left-side significant differences of chaos measured by positive largest Lyapunov exponents in schizophrenia patients compared to the control group. This might be interpreted that the neural activity during rest in schizophrenic patients is significantly more chaotic than in the control group. These data suggest that chaotic-like cognition and dissociation in patients with schizophrenia related to dysregulation in the verbal left hemisphere that display dysfunction in schizophrenia could be related to chaotic brain processes that might be a cause of random-like disorganization in mental processes. These changes in the chaotic dynamics might represent specific characteristics of dissociative states and it raises the question about a conceptual nature of the chaotic states. Important feature of chaotic transitions is a self-organization that means the spontaneous order arising in a system when certain parameters of the system reach critical values (Isaacs et al. 2003). For example, in brain simulation studies of interacting neural assemblies the abrupt switching between synchronous and stochastic random activity has been observed (Bauer and Pawelzik, 1993). These findings indicate that the cortical oscillatory activity which leads to "self-synchronization transitions" may serve as a paradigm for synchronization phenomena and a mode of self-organization in populations of interacting neurons (Kuramoto 1984; Acebron et al. 2005). These findings have a great significance because synchronization phenomena linked to integration of different neural events into a coherent whole enable mental phenomena and consciousness (Singer 2001; Lee et al. 2003).

Chapter 9

CONSCIOUSNESS EXPERIENCED BUT UNEXPLAINED

9.1. CHAOS, CONSCIOUSNESS AND CAUSALITY

According to Freeman chaos underlies the ability of the brain to respond flexibly to the outside world and to generate novel activity patterns, including those that are experienced as fresh ideas. Chaos expresses the underlying unpredictable order of attractors that could explain the complex behaviour of the brain (Freeman, 1991; 2000; 2001; Skarda and Freeman, 1987). On the psychological level these neurophysiological processes probably correspond to prototypes of intentional behaviour (neurophysiologically located in the limbic system) (Freeman, 2001). Chaos in the brain implicates the degree of unpredictability of mental and behavioral events that is in full accord with the extent of variations in the space-time patterns of the activity of chaotic systems (Freeman, 1999). The discovery of chaos has profound implications for the study of brain functions as a dynamic system that has a collection of attractors which forms an "attractor landscape" in the web of synaptic connections modified by prior learning (Skarda and Freeman, 1987) that could correspond to intentional archetypes (Freeman 2000). These pre-existing chaotic fluctuations (intentional archetypes) are enhanced by input, forcing the selection of a new macroscopic state and the attractor determines the response. The linear view proposed by stimulus-response reflex determinism is not appropriate for the dynamics that leads to nonlinear chain of cause and effect from stimulus to response that is present during chaotic brain processes (Freeman, 1999). In these chaotic self-organizing systems is "linear causality" replaced by "circular causality" that represents a concept useful for describing multilevel interactions between microscopic neurons in assemblies and the macroscopic emergent state variable that organizes them. Circular causality can serve as the framework for explaining the operation of awareness and intentional action when the multimodal macroscopic patterns converge simultaneously into the limbic system, and the results of integration over time and space are simultaneously returned to all of the sensory systems (Freeman, 1999).

These principles are expressed on the parallel psychological level where archetypes of intentional behaviour correspond to images in the mind in the process of formatting complexes from the pre-existing archetypes as ordering factors. Intentionality thus represents a key concept which enables to link neuron and brain to goal-directed behaviour through brain dynamics (Freeman, 2000). According to Freeman an archetypal form of intentional behaviour is an act of observation in space-time, by which information is sought for the guidance of future action to explore unpredictable and ever-changing environments. These acts are based in the brain dynamics that creates spatiotemporal patterns of neural activity, serving as images of goals, of command sequences by which to act to reach goals, and of expected changes in sensory input resulting from intended actions. An intentional act is completed upon modification of the system by itself through learning (Freeman, 2000). These known psychological principles may be related to nonlinear mesoscopic brain dynamics. This dynamics is linked to construction of meaningful patterns of neural activity which on the psychological level could correspond to archetypes as ordering factors of conscious and unconscious mental events and behaviour, which lead to formation of complexes (Jung, 1972a,c).

Circular processes on the neurophysiological level may correspond to psychological events that are linked to multilevel connection of dissociated contents during chaotic competition. This psychological archetypal tendency to the connection of the conflicting dissociated contents was termed by Jung as "transcendent function" (Jung, 1972) and from the neurophysiological point of view it could corresponds to chaotic nonlinear processes in the brain linked to unpredictability and generation of "fresh ideas" and corresponding novel activity patterns that enables integration of dissociated states. From the point of view of Jung's concept these self-organizing psychobiological processes may present the principal unity between the dynamic patterns of "neurophysiological circularity" and corresponding "psychological circularity" that may be supposed to be the source of mental images termed as symbols of the Self. These symbols express the psychological wholeness in the corresponding form of images of the circles and symmetric arrangements that "mirror" underlying brain functions as well as "laws" of the human psyche. These symmetric patterns are repeatedly reported in dreams, myths and religious rituals across many cultures and are connected to experienced union of psychological opposites overcoming dissociated state (Jung, 1972).

These findings support the view of the personality as a non-linear self-organized dynamic system with archetypes as pre-existing principles of organization that within the personality manifest as a psychological complex with impersonal characteristics mediated through myths and rituals or through consciousness (McDowell, 2001). From this point of view Jung's concept of the archetype and complex can be understood also in terms of current scientific research (Saunders and Skar, 2001). These connections suggest the value of cognitive neuroscience for investigating psychodynamic theory and the nature of archetypes understood on the level of primitive conceptual structures (Knox, 2001) and it corresponds to Jung's intuition about the archetype as a dynamic entity that may be expressed in mathematical terms (von Franz, 1974).

9.2. MIND AND PHYSICAL WORLD

According to Penrose's hypothesis, psychic processes and consciousness emerge non-computably from the Platonic world of mathematics by process of objective reduction. Similarly Jung (1989, p. 537) wrote: "Undoubtedly the idea of the unus mundus is founded on the assumption that the multiplicity of the empirical world rests on an underlying unity, and that not two or more fundamentally different worlds exist side by side or are mingled with one another..." Jung (1989, p. 537) thought that even the psychic world which is extraordinarily different from the physical world, does not have its roots outside the one cosmos because causal connections exist between the psyche and the body that point to their unitary nature.

Jung also thought that microphysics comes under the unknown side of matter, similarly as the psychology of complexes and archetypes is pushing forward into the unknown side of the psyche, uncovering underlying dynamics governing the human mind. According to Jung both lines of inquiry have yielded findings which can be conceived only by means of antinomies and developed concepts which display important analogies (Jung, 1989). Jung (1989) thought that if this tendency should become more pronounced in the future, the hypothesis of the unity of both disciplines would be probable. According to Jung's view the empirical reality discovered in both psychology and physics has a transcendental background that is as much physical as psychic and therefore neither, but rather a third thing, since in essence it is transcendental.

Jung thought that "...the background of our empirical world thus appears to be in fact an unus mundus. This is at least a probable hypothesis which satisfies the fundamental tenet of scientific theory: 'Explanatory principles are not to be multiplied beyond the necessary.' The transcendental psychophysical background corresponds to a 'potential world' in so far as all those conditions which determine the form of empirical phenomena are inherent in it. This obviously holds good as much for physics as for psychology,..." (1989, p. 537). The epistemological views of both authors Jung and Penrose are very similar. According to Jung the theory of archetypes is analogical to the "Platonic world" of psychic existence in which psychic contents and complexes originate in the archetypal background (von Franz, 1964, 1974). Similarly Penrose postulated that quantum-gravity processes in the brain lead to a reduction and expression of "Platonic idea" into the world of things by the objective reduction in the brain. The reduction enables to create inner psychological order, similarly as external world of things and other cosmological events are created. Jung and Penrose using the modern language of science have expressed an old philosophical and epistemological idea that everything has two principles that explain its being as essence and existence.

Whether mathematical knowledge is only an idealization of the external world or represents an essence of the physical world is an open question of science. The dominate paradigm in psychology and neuroscience at this time is neuronal materialism, although modern physics includes findings that lead to a substantial revision of our opinion about space and time. When we think of the complexity of the human mind and brain functions, it might be necessary to consider that modern mathematics and physics in their applications in the field of neuroscience may substantially change our understanding of mind and brain. For example, nonlinear mathematics and chaos theory in the field of neuroscience potentially could explain brain complexity and interactions among neural assemblies. Because there is no rigorous border for (classical and quantum) chaotic fluctuations it is possible to suppose that the mental state related to quantum fluctuations may induce chaotic self-organization on neural or other hierarchical levels of living organism with fractal structure (Basar and Guntekin, 2006; Courtial and Bailon-Moreno, 2006; King, 1991, 1997). From this point of view ultimate level of chaotic self-organization might originate in the process of wave function collapse that may cause the chaotic process of "creating information". This concept could potentially be supportive for objective evidence for the existence of consciousness as an entity "beyond" its neural correlates and its possible archetypal demonstration related to quantum phenomena (Kutner and Rosenblum, 2006).

These preliminary findings may provide empirical link for further research regarding connections between quantum level and chaotic self-organization related to mental processes. Chaotic transitions probably emerge in a wide variety of cognitive phenomena and likely reflect also the parallel, hierarchical and divided (or dissociated) structure of the mind (Bob, 2003b; Faure and Korn, 2001). According to Putnam (1997), retrieval of a dissociated mental state may lead to rapid changes in mood and behavior. Specific characteristics of these changes may be chaotic shifts in neural dynamics with extreme sensitivity at the initial phase of the mental process (Putnam, 1997; Bob, 2003b) that can be assessed by nonlinear analysis of EEG or other psychophysiological measures such as electrodermal activity (Bob, 2007a; Bob et al., 2007b,c). For example, increased chaoticity of electrodermal activity during hypnotic recall of dissociated traumatic memories from early childhood has been observed (Bob, 2007a).

Werner Heisenberg thought that a revival of the Aristotelian concept of potentia was important for understanding of quantum physics because quantum entities did not possess positions and momenta but rather the potentiality for such properties when they were actually measured (Heisenberg, 1958; Wheeler, and Zurek, 1983). The category of "potentiality" may represent a useful analogy for the neurobiological approach to consciousness. Consciousness from this point of view may be understood not only as an artifact of biological processes but as a complementary part of the material world of things. Accordingly, the mind as a self-organizing component of the neural system is linked to fundamental physical processes of self-organization within the nature and cosmos. This philosophical view extends the term complementarity defined by Niels Bohr as a concept that a single model may not be adequate to explain all the observations made of atomic or subatomic systems in different experiments (Isaacs, Daintith, and Martin, 2003; Wheeler, and Zurek, 1983), which implicates wave-particle duality for description of quantum phenomena. Similarly, the complementarity and duality between the self-organization as analogue of Aristoteles' causa formalis and chemical and subatomic structures as analogue of causa materialis are necessary needed for description and understanding of brain organization and living structures. The complementarity between self-organizing mind and biological systems of the body may represent important postulate for psychosomatic processes, which show that disordered self-organized mind leads to illnesses of the body and on the other hand that destructive influences from the outside world disturb the mind and body self-organization. These processes might represent macroscopic analogue to objective (spontaneous wave collapse) or subjective reduction (caused by interaction with the outside world). From this point of view the complementarity principle for description of psychological and physical disorders is needed and represent necessary paradigm for medical science and practice.

Mathematical realism in the theory of relativity and quantum mechanics negotiates naive realism and shows our seeing of the world as a special case of more general mathematical and physical laws. Similarly applications of chaos theory in psychology and neuroscience and also first theoretical and empirical studies focused on applications of quantum theory in neurobiological systems represent new paradigm for the study of consciousness with a great heuristic value which may uncover new understanding of the human mind.

According to this concept the Platonic mathematical world incarnates into the physical world of objects as well as into the contents of the human mind. On general level these findings suggest that the so-called "brain centered" theories are not necessary for further study of consciousness (Tonneau, 2004) and underlying physical processes important for consciousness in principle must not be included within existing neurophysiological concepts of the brain processes.

REFERENCES

Acebron, J.A., Bonilla, L.L, Perez, C.J., Ritort, F., Spigler, R. (2005). The Kuramoto model: a simple paradigm for synchronization phenomena. *Reviews of Modern Physics, 77*, 137-185.

Adamec, R.E. (1990). Does kindling model anything clinically relevant? *Biological Psychiatry, 27*, 249-79.

Adamec, R. (1997). Transmitter systems involved in neural plasticity underlying increased anxiety and defense-implications for understanding anxiety following traumatic stress. *Neuroscience and Biobehavioral Reviews, 21*, 755-65.

Adamec, R.E. (1999). Evidence that limbic neural plasticity in the right hemisphere mediates partial kindling induced lasting increases in anxiety-like behavior: effects of low frequency stimulation (Quenching?) on long-term potentiation of amygdala efferents and behavior following kindling. *Brain Research, 839*, 133-152.

Adamec, R.E. and McKay, D. (1993). Amygdala kindling, anxiety, and corticotopin releasing factor (CRF). *Physiology and Behavior, 54*, 423-431.

Agargun, M.Y., Tekeoglu, I., Kara, H., Adak, B., and Ercan, M. (1998). Hypnotizability, pain threshold, and dissociative experiences. *Biological Psychiatry, 44*, 66-71.

Ahern, G.L., Herring, A.M., Tackenberg, J., and Seeger, J.F. (1993). The association of multiple personality and temporolimbic epilepsy: Intracarotid amobarbital test observations. *Archives of Neurology, 50*, 1020-1025.

Aks, D.J. and Sprott, J. C. (2003). Resolving perceptual ambiguity in the Necker Cube: A dynamical systems approach. *Journal of Non-linear Dynamics in Psychology and the Life Sciences, 7*, 159-178.

Alarcon, G., Binnie, C.D., Elwes, R.D., and Polkey, C.E. (1995). Power spectrum and intracranial EEG patterns at seizure onset in partial epilepsy. *Electroencephalography and Clinical Neurophysiology, 94*, 326-337.

Albright, P.S. and Burnham, B.M. (1980). Development of a new pharmacological seizure model: Effects of anticonvulsants on cortical and amygdala-kindled seizures in the rats. *Epilepsia, 21*, 681-689.

Alison, R.B. (1974). A new treatment approach for multiple personalities. *American Journal of Clinical Hypnosis, 17*, 15-32.

Allen, P.J., Fish, D.R., and Smith, S.J. (1992). Very high-frequency rhythmic activity during SEEG suppression in frontal lobe epilepsy. *Electroencephalography and Clinical Neurophysiology, 82*, 155-159.

Alvarez, J. (2001). Neural hypersynchronization, creativity and endogenous psychoses. *Medical Hypotheses, 56*, 672-685.

American Psychiatric Association (1980). A psychiatric glossary, 5th ed. Washington, DC: Author.

American Psychiatric Association (1987). DSM III-R, Diagnostic and Statistical Manual of Mental Disorders. Fourth Edition. Washington DC: American Psychiatric Association.

American Psychiatric Association (1994). DSM IV, Diagnostic and Statistical Manual of Mental Disorders. Fourth Edition. Washington DC: American Psychiatric Association, 1994.

Andersen, E. (1986). Peiraqueductal gray and cerebral cortex modulate responses of medial thalamic neurons to noxious stimulation. *Brain Research, 375*, 30-36.

Anderson, C.M., Teicher, M.H., Polcari, A., and Renshaw, P.F. (2002). Abnormal T2 relaxation time in the cerebellar vermis of adults sexually abused in childhood: potential role of the vermis in stress-enhanced risk for drug abuse. *Psychoneuroendocrinology, 27*, 231–44.

Andreasen, N.C., Arndt, S., Alliger, R., Miller, D., and Flaum, M. (1995). Symptoms of schizophrenia. Methods, meanings, and mechanisms. *Archives of General Psychiatry, 52*, 341–351

Arp, R. (2005). Selectivity, integration, and the psycho-neuro-biological continuum. *Journal of Mind and Behavior, 26*, 35-64.

Atmanspacher, H. and Fach, W. (2005). Acategoriality as mental instability. *Journal of Mind and Behavior, 26*, 181-205.

Avnon, Y., Nitzan, M., Sprecher, E., Rogowski, Z., and Yarnitsky, D. (2004). Autonomic asymmetry in migraine: augmented parasympathetic activation in left unilateral migraineurs. *Brain, 127*, 2099-2108.

Baars, B.J. (1988). A Cognitive Theory of Consciousness. Cambridge: Cambridge University Press.

Baars, B.J. (1997). Some essential differences between consciousness and attention, perception, and working memory. *Consciousness and Cognition, 6*, 363–371.

Baars, B.J. (1999). Attention versus consciousness in the visual brain: differences in conception, phenomenology, behaviour, neuroanatomy, and physiology. *Journal of General Psychology, 12*, 224–233.

Baars, B. J. (2002). The conscious access hypothesis: origins and recent evidence. *Trends in Cognitive Sciences, 6*, 47-52.

Badura, A.S., Reiter, R.C., Altmaier, E.M., Rhomberg, A., and Elsa, D. (1997). Dissociation, somatization, substance abuse, and coping in women with chronic pelvic pain. *Obstetrics and Gynecology, 90*, 405–10.

Bantick, S.J., Wise, R.G., Ploghaus, A., Clare, S., Smith, S.M., and Tracey, I. (2002). Imaging how attention modulates pain in humans using functional MRI. *Brain, 125*, 310-9.

Bao AM, Meynen G, Swaab DF (2008). The stress system in depression and neurodegeneration: Focus on the human hypothalamus. *Brain Research Reviews, 57,* 531-53.

Baron, R., Baron, Y., Disbrow, E., and Roberts, T.P. (1999). Brain processing of capsaicin-induced secondary hyperalgesia: a functional MRI study. *Neurology, 53,* 548-57.

Barton, S. (1994). Chaos, self-organization, and psychology. *American Psychologist, 49,* 5-14.

Barrera-Mera, B. and Barrera-Calva, E. (1998). The Cartesian clock metaphor for pineal gland operation pervades the origin of modern chronobiology. *Neuroscience and Biobehavioral Reviews, 23,* 1-4.

Barret, D. (1994). Dreams in dissociative disorders. *Dreaming, 4,* 165-175.

Barret, D. (1995). The dream character as prototype for the multiple personality alter. *Dissociation 8,* 66-68.

Barret, D. (1996). Dreams in multiple personality disorder. In D. Barret (Ed.), *Trauma and dreams* (pp. 68-81). Harvard University Press.

Barry, E., Sussman, N.M., Bosley, T.M., and Harner, R.N. (1985). Ictal blindness and status epilepticus amauroticus. *Epilepsia, 26,* 577-84.

Basar, E., and Guntekin, B. (2007). A breakthrough in neuroscience needs a "Nebulous Cartesian System" Oscillations, quantum dynamics and chaos in the brain and vegetative system. *International Journal of Psychophysiology, 64,* 108-122.

Bath, K.G. and Lee, F.S. (2006). Variant BDNF (Val66Met) impact on brain structure and function. *Cognitive Affective and Behavioral Neuroscience, 6,* 79-85.

Bauer, H.U. and Pawelzik, K. (1993). Alternating oscillatory and stochastic dynamics in a model for a neuronal assembly. *Physica D, 69,* 380-393.

Bauer, R.M. (1998). Physiological measures of emotions. *Journal of Clinical Neurophysiology, 15,* 388-396.

Baumgartner, C., Lurge R,S., and Leutmezer, F. (2001). Autonomic symptoms during epileptic seizures. *Epileptic Disorders, 3,* 103-116.

Baydas, G., Ozveren, F., Akdemir, I., Tuzcu, M., and Yasar, A. (2005). Learning and memory deficits in rats induced by chronic thinner exposure are reversed by melatonin. *Journal of Pineal Research, 39,* 50-6.

Bechara A., Tranel, D., Damasio, H., Adolphs, R., Rockland, C., and Damasio, A.R. (1995). Double dissociation of conditioning and declarative knowledge relative to the amygdala and hippocampus in humans. *Science, 269,* 1115-1118.

Beck, A.T., Rush, A.J., Shaw, B.F., and Emery, G. (1979). *Cognitive therapy of depression.* New York: Willey.

Beck, A. T., Steer, R. A., and Brown, G. K. (1996). Manual for Beck Depression Inventory-II. San Antonio, TX: Psychological Corporation.

Beck, F., and Eccles, J.C. (1992). Quantum aspects of brain activity and the role of consciousness. *Proceedings of the National Academy of Sciences of the United States of America, 89,* 11357-11361.

Benson, D. F. (1986). Interictal behaviour disorders in epilepsy. *Psychiatric Clinics of North America, 9,* 283-292.

Benson, F., Miller, B.L., and Signer, S.F. (1986). Dual personality associated with epilepsy. *Archives of Neurology, 43*, 471-474.

Berkhout, J., Walter, D.O., and Adey, W.R. (1969). Alteration of the Human Electroencephalogram Induced by Stressful Verbal Activity. *Electroencephalography and clinical Neurophysiology, 27*, 457-469.

Bernat, E., Bunce, S., and Shevrin, H. (2001). Event-related brain potentials differentiate positive and negative mood adjectives during both supraliminal and subliminal visual processing. *International Journal of Psychophysiology, 42*, 11-34.

Bernstein, E.M. and Putnam, F.W. (1986). Development, Reliability, and Validity of a Dissociation Scale. *Journal of Nervous and Mental Disease, 174*, 727-735.

Binder, D.K. and Scharfman, H.E. (2004). Brain-derived neurotrophic factor. *Growth Factors, 22*, 123-31.

Birbaumer, N., Flor, H., Lutzenberger, W., and Elbert, T. (1995). Chaos and order in the human brain. *Electroencephalography and Clinical Neurophysiolology, Suppl. 44*, 450-459.

Blake, R., Yu, K., Lokey, M. and Norman, H. (1998). Binocular rivalry and motion perception. *Journal of Cognitive Neuroscience, 10*, 46–60.

Blanke, O., Ortigue, S., Landis, T., and Seeck, M. (2002). Neuropsychology: Stimulating illusory own-body perceptions. *Nature, 419*, 269-270.

Bleuler, E. (1918/1906). Consciousness and association. Eder, M. D. (trans.). In C. G. Jung (Ed.), *Studies in word-association* (pp. 266-296). London: William Heinemann.

Bleuler, E. (1911/1955). *Dementia praecox or the group of the schizophrenias.* New York: International University Press.

Bleuler, E. (1924). *Textbook of Psychiatry.* A.A Brill (trans.). New York: Macmillan Publishing Co. Inc.

Bliss, E.L. (1980). Multiple personalities. A report of 14 cases with implications for schizophrenia and hysteria. *Archives of General Psychiatry, 37*, 1388-97.

Blumer, D., Wakhlu, S., Davies, K., and Hermann, B. (1998). Psychiatric outcome of temporal lobectomy for epilepsy: incidence and treatment of psychiatric complications. *Epilepsia, 39*, 478 –86.

Boatright, J.H., Rubim, N.M., and Iuvone, P.M. (1994). Regulation of endogenous dopamine release in amphibian retina by melatonin: the role of GABA. *Visual Neuroscience, 11*, 1013–1018.

Bob, P. (2003a). Subliminal processes dissociation and the 'I'. *Journal of Analytical Psychology, 48*, 307-316.

Bob, P. (2003b). Dissociation and Neuroscience: History and New Perspectives. *International Journal of Neuroscience, 113*, 903-914.

Bob, P. (2004). Dissociative processes, multiple personality and dream functions. *American Journal of Psychotherapy, 58*, 139-149.

Bob, P. (2004b). Perinatal hypoxia and brain disorders. *Neurology, Psychiatry and Brain Research, 11*, 77-82.

Bob, P. (2004c). Psychophysiology of hypnotic abreaction. *Homeostasis in Health and Disease, 43*, 109-111.

Bob., P. (2006). The chaotic brain, dissociative states, and dream function. *ReVision, 29*, 20-27.

Bob, P. (2007a). Chaotic patterns of electrodermal activity during dissociated state released by hypnotic abreaction. *International Journal of Clinical and Experimental Hypnosis, 55*, 435-436.

Bob, P. (2007b). Consciousness and co-consciousness, binding problem and schizophrenia. *Neuroendocrinology Letters, 28*, 723-6.

Bob, P. (2007c). Dissociation, forced normalization and dynamic multi-stability of the brain. *Neuroendocrinology Letters, 28*, 231-246.

Bob, P. (2008). Pain, dissociation and subliminal self-representations. *Consciousness and Cognition, 17*, 355-369.

Bob, P. (2008b). Quantum Science and the Nature of Mind. *Journal of Mind and Behavior* (in press).

Bob, P., Susta, M., Pavlat, J., Hynek, K., and Raboch, J. (2005). Depression, traumatic dissociation and epileptic-like phenomena. *Neuroendocrinology letters, 26*, 321-325.

Bob P, Glaslova K, Susta M, Jasova D, and Raboch J. (2006a). Traumatic dissociation, epileptic-like phenomena, and schizophrenia. *Neuroendocrinology Letters, 27*, 321-6.

Bob, P., Kukleta, M., Riecansky, I., Susta, M., Kukumberg, P., and Jagla, F. (2006b). Chaotic EEG patterns during recall of stressfull memory related to panic attack. *Physiological Research, 55* (Suppl 1), 113-119.

Bob, P., Susta, M., Prochazkova-Vecerova, A., Kukleta, M., Pavlat, J., Jagla, F., Raboch J. (2006). Limbic irritability and chaotic neural response during conflicting stroop task in the patients with unipolar depression. *Physiological Research 55* Suppl 1, S107-12.

Bob, P., Kukleta, M., Jagla, F. (2007a). Traumatic stress, anxiety and epilepsy. *Studia Psychologica, 49*, 127-133.

Bob, P., Susta, M., Chladek, J., Glaslova, K., Fedor-Freybergh, P. (2007b). Neural complexity, dissociation and schizophrenia. *Medical Science Monitor, 13*, 1-5.

Bob, P., Chladek, J., Susta, M., Glaslova, K., Jagla, F., Kukleta, M. (2007c). Neural chaos and schizophrenia. *General Physiology and Biophysics, 26*, 298-305.

Bob, P., Susta, M., Glaslova, K., Pavlat, J., and Raboch, J. (2007d). Lateralized electrodermal dysfunction and complexity in patients with schizophrenia and depression. *Neuroendocrinology Letters, 28*, 11-5.

Bob, P., Susta, M., Glaslova, K., Fedor-Freybergh, P., Pavlat, J., Miklosko, J., and Raboch, J. (2007e). Dissociation, epileptic-like activity and lateralized electrodermal dysfunction in patients with schizophrenia and depression. *Neuroendocrinology letters, 28*, 868-74.

Bob, P. and Fedor-Freybergh, P. (2008). Melatonin, consciousness and traumatic stress. *Journal of Pineal Research, 44*, 341-347.

Bob, P. Siroka, I., Susta, M. (2008). Chaotic patterns of autonomic activity during hypnotic recall. *International Journal of Neuroscience, 118*, (in press).

Bobes, M.A., Lopera, F., Garcia, M., Diaz-Comas, L., Galan, L., and Valdes-Sosa, M. (2003). Covert matching of unfamiliar faces in a case of prosopagnosia: an ERP study. *Cortex, 39*, 41-56.

Bogen, J.E. and Bogen, G.M. (1969). The other side of the brain: III. The corpus callosum and creativity. *Bulletin of Los Angeles Neurological Society, 34*, 191-220.

Boksa, P. and El-Khodor, B.F. (2003). Birth insult interacts with stress at adulthood to alter dopaminergic function in animal models: possible implications for schizophrenia and other disorders. *Neuroscience Biobehavioral Reviews, 27*, 91-101.

Boleloucky, Z. (1986). Multiple, dissociated personality- new interest in an old problem. *Ceskoslovenska Psychiatrie, 82*, 318- 327.

Bornhovd, K., Quante, M., Glauche, V., Bromm, B., Weiller, C., and Buchel, C. (2002). Painful stimuli evoke different stimulus-response functions in the amygdala, prefrontal, insula and somatosensory cortex: a single trial fMRI study. *Brain, 125*, 1326-36.

Bottero, A. (2001). A history of dissociative schizophrenia. *L' Evolution Psychiatrique, 66*, 43-60.

Bovensiepen, G. (2006). Attachment-dissociation network: some thoughts about a modern complex theory. *Journal of Analytical Psychology, 51*, 451-66.

Bower, G.H. (1981). Mood and Memory. *American Psychologist, 36*, 129-148.

Bowers, M. K. and Brecher, S. (1955). The emergence of multiple personalities in the course of hypnotic investigation. *International Journal of Clinical and Experimental Hypnosis, 3*, 188-199.

Bowman, E.S. and Coons, P.M. (2000). The differential diagnosis of epilepsy, pseudoseizures, dissociative identity disorder, and dissociative disorder not otherwise specified. *Bulletin of the Menninger Clinic, 64*, 164-180.

Braitenberg, V. (1978). Cell assemblies in the cerebral cortex. In R.Heim and G. Palm (Eds.) Theoretical approaches to complex systems. *Lecture notes in biomathematics, 21*, (pp. 171–188). Berlin: Springer.

Bramham, C.R. and Messaoudi, E. (2005). BDNF function in adult synaptic plasticity: the synaptic consolidation hypothesis. *Progress in Neurobiology, 76*, 99-125.

Brandeis, D. and Lehmann, D. (1986). Event-related potentials of the brain and cognitive processes: approaches and applications. *Neuropsychologia, 24*, 151-68.

Braun, B.G. (1986). Issues in the psychotherapy of multiple personality disorder. In Braun BG, editor. *Treatment of multiple personality disorder*. Washington, DC: American Psychiatric Press, pp. 1-28,.

Brazdil, M., Rektor, I., Daniel, P., Dufek, M., and Jurak, P. (2001). Intracerebral event-related potentials to subthreshold target stimuli. *Clinical Neurophysiology, 112*, 650-61.

Breakspear, M. (2006). The nonlinear theory of schizophrenia. *Australian and New Zealand Journal of Psychiatry, 40*, 20-35.

Bremner, J.D., Randall, P., Scott, T. M., Bronen, R. A., Seibyl, J. P., Southwick, S. M., Delaney, R. C., and Charney, D. S. (1995). MRI-based measurement of hippocampal volume in combat-related posttraumatic stress disorder. *American Journal of Psychiatry, 152*, 973-981.

Bremner, J.D. (2006). The relationship between cognitive and brain changes in posttraumatic stress disorder. *Annals of the New York Academy of Sciences, 1071*, 80-6.

Brende, J.O. (1982). Electrodermal responses in posttraumatic syndromes. A pilot study of cerebral hemisphere functioning in Vietnam veterans. *Journal of Nervous and Mental Disease, 170*, 352-361.

Brende, J. O. (1984). The psychophysiologic manifestations of dissociation: Electrodermal responses in a multiple personality patient. *Psychiatric Clinics of North America, 7*, 41-50.

Brenner, I. (1996). The characterological basis of multiple personality. *American Journal of Psychotherapy, 52*, 154-66.

Brenner, I. (1999). Deconstructing DID. *American Journal of Psychotherapy, 53*, 344-360.

Brenner, I. (2001). *Dissociation of trauma: Theory, phenomenology and technique.* Boston: International Universities Press.

Bressler, S.L., Coppola, R., and Nakamura, R. (1993). Episodic multiregional cortical coherence at multiple frequencies during visual task performance. *Nature , 366*, 153–156.

Breuer, J. and Freud, S. (1895). *Studies in hysteria.* New York: Basic Books.

Brewin, C.R. and Andrews, B. (1998). Recovered memories of trauma: Phenomenology and cognitive mechanisms. *Clinical Psychology Review, 18*, 949-970.

Brewin, C.R. Autobiographical memory for trauma: update on four controversies. *Memory* 2007, 15, 227-48.

Briere, J. and Conte, J. (1989). Amnesia and adults molested as children: Testing theories of repression. Paper presented at the 97th Annual Convention of the American Psychological Association, New Orleans.

Briere, J. (1996). Psychometric review of the Trauma Symptom Checklist-40, In B.H. Stamm, (Ed.), *Measurement of stress, trauma, and adaptation.* Lutherville: Sidran Press.

Briquet, P. (1859). *Traité clinique et therapeutique de l'hystérie.* Paris: JB Baillière

Brown, B.G. (1984). Towards a Theory of Multiple Personality and Other Dissociative Phenomena. *Psychiatric Clinics of North America, 7*, 171-193.

Brown, D. and Fromm, E. (1986). *Hypnotherapy and hypnoanalysis.* Hillsdale, NJ: L. Erlbaum Associates.

Brown, R., Kocsis, J.H., Caroff, S., Amsterdam, J., Winokur, A., Stokes, P.E., Frazer, A. (1985). Differences in nocturnal melatonin secretion between melancholic depressed patients and control subjects. *American Journal of Psychiatry, 142*, 811–816.

Brown, R.J. and Trimble, M.R. (2000). Dissociative psychopathology, non-epileptic seizures, and neurology. *Journal of Neurology, Neurosurgery and Psychiatry, 69*, 285-9.

Bunge, S.A., Ochsner, K.N., Reskond, J.E., Glover, G.H., and Gabrieli, J.D.E. (2001). Prefrontal regions involved in keeping information in and out of mind. *Brain, 124*, 2074-86.

Butler, L.D., Duran, R.E.F., Jasiukaitis, P., Koopman, CH. and Spiegel, D. (1996). Hypnotizability and Traumatic Experience: A Diathesis-Stress Model of Dissociative Symptomatology. *American Journal of Psychiatry, Festschrift Supplement, 153*, 42-62.

Bystritsky, A., Leuchter, A.F., and Vapnik T. (1999). EEG abnormalities in nonmedicated panic disorder. *Journal of Nervous and Mental Disease, 187*, 113-4.

Cadell, S., Regehr, C., and Hemsworth, D. (2003). Factors contributing to posttraumatic growth: a proposed structural equation model. *American Journal of Orthopsychiatry, 73*, 279-88.

Cahill, L. (1997). The neurobiology of emotionally influenced memory. Implications for understanding traumatic memory. *Annals of the New York Academy of Sciences, 821*, 238-46.

Cahill, L. and McGaugh, J.L. (1998). Mechanisms of emotional arousal and lasting declarative memory. *Trends in Neurosciences, 21*, 294-9.

Callaway, C. W., Lydic, R., Baghdoyan, H. A., and Hobson, J. A. (1987). Pontogeniculooccipital waves: Spontaneous visual system activity during rapid eye movement sleep. *Cellular and Molecular Neurobiology, 7*, 105-109.

Casey, K.L. (1999). Forebrain mechanisms of nociception and pain: analysis through imaging. *Proceedings of the National Academy of Sciences of the United States of America, 96*, 7668– 7674.

Cerullo, A., Tinupe, P., Provini, F., Contin, M., Rosati, A., Marini, C., and Cortelli, P. (1998). Autonomic and hormonal ictal changes in gelastic seizures from hypothalamic hamartomas. *Electroencephalography and Clinical Neurophysiology, 107*, 317-322.

Chapman, C. R. and Nakamura, Y. (1999). A passion of the soul: an introduction to pain for consciousness researchers. *Consciousness and Cognition, 8*, 391-422.

Chaudhury, D., Wang, L.M., and Colwell, C.S. (2005). Circadian regulation of hippocampal long-term potentiation. *Journal Biological Rhythms, 20*, 225–236.

Chaplin, J., Yepez, R. and Shorvon, S. (1990). A quantitative approach to measuring the social effects of epilepsy. *Neuroepidemiology, 9*, 151–158.

Chatrian, G.E., Bergamini, L., Dondey, M., et al. (1974). A glossary of terms most commonly used by clinical electroencephalographers. *Electroencephalography and Clinical Neurophysiology, 37*, 538-548.

Cheek, D. B. (1959). Unconscious perception of meaningful sounds during surgical anesthesia as revealed under hypnosis. *American Journal of Clinical Hypnosis, 7*, 55-59.

Cheek, D. B. (1964). Surgical memory and reaction to careless conversation. *American Journal of Clinical Hypnosis, 6*, 237-40.

Cheek, D. B. (1964). Further evidence of persistence of hearing under chemo-anestezia: detailed case report. *American Journal of Clinical Hypnosis, 7*, 55-59.

Cheek, D. B. (1966). The meaning of continued hearing sense under general chemo-anestezia: A progress report and report of a case. *American Journal of Clinical Hypnosis, 8*, 275-280.

Chen, A,C. (2001). New perspectives in EEG/MEG brain mapping and PET/fMRI neuroimaging of human pain. *International Journal of Psychophysiology, 42*, 147-59.

Chertok, L., Michaux, D., and Droin, M.C. (1977). Dynamics of hypnotic analgesia: some new data. *Journal of Nervous and Mental Disease, 164*, 88-96.

Chu, J. and Dill, D. (1990). Dissociative Symptoms in Relation to Chidhood Sexual and Physical Abuse. *American Journal of Psychiatry, 147*, 887-892.

Coghill, R.C., Sang, C.N., Maisog, J.M., and Iadarola, M.J. (1999). Pain intensity processing within the human brain: a bilateral, distributed mechanism. *Journal of Neurophysiology, 82*, 1934-1943.

Coghill, R.C., McHaffie, J.G., and Yen, Y.-F. (2003). Neural correlates of interindividual differences in the subjective experience of pain. *Proceedings of the National Academy of Sciences of the United States of America, 100*, 8538– 8542.

Condes-Lara, M., Omana-Zapata, I., Leon-Olea, M., and Sanchez-Alvarez, M. (1989). Dorsal raphe and nociceptive stimulations evoke convergent responses on the thalamic centralis lateralis and medial prefrontal cortex neurons. *Brain Research, 499,* 145-52.

Coons, P.M. (1980). Multiple personality: diagnostic considerations. *Journal of Clinical Psychiatry, 41,* 330-36.

Coons, P.M., Milstein, V., and Marley, C. (1982). EEG studies of two multiple personality and a control. *Archives of General Psychiatry, 39,* 823-825.

Coons, P.M., Bowman, E.S., and Milstein, V. (1988). Multiple personality disorder. A clinical investigation of 50 cases. *Journal of Nervous and Mental Disease, 176,* 519-27.

Coons, P. M., Bowman E.S., and Pellow T.A. (1989). Post-traumatic aspects of the treatment of victims of sexual abuse and incest. *Psychiatric Clinics of North America, 12,* 325-327.

Coleman-Mensches, K. and McGaugh, J.L. (1995). Differential involvement of the right and left amygdalae in expression of memory for aversively motivated training. *Brain Research 670,* 75-81.

Colman, A.M. (2003). *A Dictionary of Psychology.* New York: Oxford University Press.

Corcoran, C., Walker, E., Huot, R., Mittal, V., Tessner, K., Kestler, L., and Malaspina, D. (2003). The stress cascade and schizophrenia: etiology and onset. *Schizophrenia Bulletin, 29,* 671-92.

Corkin, S. and Hebben N. (1981). Subjective estimates of chronic pain before and after psychosurgery or treatment in a pain unit (Abstract). *Pain, Suppl. 1,* S150.

Courtial, J.P. and Bailon-Moreno, R. (2006). The structure of scientific knowledge and a fractal model of thought. *Journal of Mind and Behavior, 27,* 149-165.

Coveney, P. and Highfield, R. (1996). *Frontiers of Complexity.* London: Faber and Faber.

Craig, A.D. (2001). The neural representations of the physiological condition of the body: Pain as an aspect of homeostasis. *Journal of Physiology, 536,* 93.

Craig, A.D. (2002). How do you feel? Interoception: the sense of the physiological condition of the body. Nature Reviews. *Neuroscience, 3,* 655-666.

Craig, A.D. (2003). A new view of pain as a homeostatic emotion. *Trends in Neurosciences, 26,* 303-7.

Crawford, H.J. (1994). Brain dynamics and hypnosis. *International Journal of Clinical and Experimental Hypnosis, 42,* 204-232.

Crick, F. (1994). *The astonishing hypothesis. The scientific search for the soul.* London: Simon and Schuster.

Crick, F. and Clark, J. (1994). "The astonishing hypothesis" An interview. *Journal of Consciousness Studies, 1* (1), 17-24.

Crick, F. and Koch, C. (2003). A framework for consciousness. *Nature Neuroscience, 6,* 119-26.

Crick, F. and Koch, C. (1992). The problem of consciousness. *Scientific American, 267*(3), 153-159.

Crick, F., and Koch, C. (1995). Are we aware of neural activity in primary visual cortex? *Nature, 375,* 121-123.

Critchley, H.D. (2002). Electrodermal Responses: What Happens in the Brain. *Neuroscientist, 8,* 132-142.

Croft, P. (2000). Testing for tenderness: what's the point? *Journal of Rheumatology, 27,* 2531– 2533.

Dalby, M.A. (1975). Behavioral effects of carbamazepine. In: *Complex partial seizures and their treatment, Advances in Neurology vol II.* Penry J.K., Daly D.D. (eds), Raven Press: New York, 331-343.

Dalgleish, T. and Power, M.J. (2004). The I of the storm-relations between self and conscious emotion experience: comment on Lambie and Marcel: *Psychological Review* 2002, 111, 812-8; discussion , 818-9.

Dawson, K.A. (2004). Temporal organization of the brain: neurocognitive mechanisms. *Brain and Cognition, 54,* 75-94.

Dawson ME, Shell AM, and Filion DL (2000). The electrodermal system. In: Cacioppo JT, Tassinary LG, Bernston GC, editors. *Handbook of Psychophysiology* (pp 200-23). Cambridge, MA: Cambridge University Press.

Dawson, M.E. and Schell, A. M. (2002). What does electrodermal activity tell us about prognosis in the schizophrenia spectrum? *Schizophrenia Research, 54,* 87-93.

Debiec, J., Doyere, V., Nader, K., and LeDoux, J.E. (2006). Directly reactivated, but not indirectly reactivated, memories undergo reconsolidation in the amygdala. *Proceedings of the National Academy of Sciences of the United States of America, 103,* 9, 3428-3433.

Debiec, J., LeDoux, J.E., and Nader, K. (2002). Cellular and Systems Reconsolidation in the Hippocampus. *Neuron, 36,* 527-38.

Derbyshire, S.W.G., Jones, A.K.P., Devani, P., Friston, K.J., Feinmann, C., Harris, M., Pearce, S., Watson, J.D.G., and Frackowiak, R.S.J. (1994). Cerebral responses to pain in patients with atypical facial pain measured by positron emission tomography. Journal of *Neurolology Neurosurgery and Psychiatry, 57,* 1166– 1172.

Derbyshire, S.W.G., Jones, A.K.P., Gyulai, F., Clark, S., Townsend, D., and Firestone, L. (1997). Pain processing during three levels of noxious stimulation produces differential patterns of central activity. *Pain, 73,* 431– 445.

Derbyshire, S.W.G. (2000). Exploring the pain ''neuromatrix''. *Current Review of Pain, 6,* 467–477.

Derbyshire, S.W.G., Jones, A.K.P., Creed, F., Starz, T., Meltzer, C.C., Townsend, D.W., Peterson, A.M., and Firestone, L. (2002). Cerebral responses to noxious thermal stimulation in chronic low back pain patients and normal controls. *Neuroimage, 16,* 158– 168.

Derbyshire, S.W.G., Whalley, M.G., Stenger, A., and Oakley, D.A. (2004). Cerebral activation during hypnotically induced and imagined pain. *Neuroimage, 23,* 392-401.

Desimone, R. and Duncan, J. (1995). Neural mechanisms of selective visual attention. *Annual Review of Neuroscience, 18,* 193–222.

Devinsky, O. (2004). Effects of seizures on autonomic and cardiovascular function. *Epilepsy Currents, 4,* 43-46.

Dewaraja, R. and Sasaki, Y. (1990). A left to right callosal transfer deficit of nonlinguistic information in alexithymia. *Psychotherapy and Psychosomatics 54,* 201-207.

Diamond, D.M., and Rose, G.M. (1994). Stress impairs LTP and hippocampal-dependent memory. *Annals of the New York Academy of Sciences, 746,* 411-414.

Dokoumetzidis, A., Iliadin, A., Macheras, P. (2001). Nonlinear dynamics and chaos theory: Concepts and applications relevant to pharmacodynamics. *Pharmacological Research, 18*, 415–426.

Dreifuss, F. (1981). Proposal for revised clinical and electroencephalographic classification of epileptic seizures. *Epilepsia, 22*, 489-501.

Duch, W. (2005). Brain-inspired conscious computing architecture. *Journal of Mind and Behavior, 26*, 1-21.

Ebrinc, S. (2002). Hypnotizability, pain threshold and dissociative experiences. *European Neuropsychopharmacology, 12* (Suppl.), 427-428.

Eccleston, C. and Crombez, G. (1999). Pain demands attention: A cognitive-affective model of the interruptive function of pain. *Psychological Bulletin, 125*, 356-366.

Edwards, H.E., MacLusky, N.J., and Burnham, W.M. (2000). The effect of seizures and kindling on reproductive hormones in the rat. *Neuroscience and Biobehavioral Reviews 24*, 753-62.

Egner, T., Jamieson, G., and Gruzelier, J. (2005). Hypnosis decouples cognitive control from conflict monitoring processes of the frontal lobe. *Neuroimage, 27*, 969-978.

Eimer, M. (2000). Event-related brain potentials distinguish processing stages involved in face perception and recognition. *Clinical Neurophysiology, 111*, 694-705.

Eisenberg, N.I., Lieberman, M.D., and Williams, K.D. (2003). Does rejection hurt: an fMRI study of social exclusion. *Science, 302*, 290-292.

Eisenberg, N.I. and Lieberman, M.D. (2004). Why rejection hurts: a common neural alarm system for physical and social pain. *Trends in Cognitive Sciences, 8*, 294-300.

Elazar, Z., and Hobson, J. A. (1985). Neuronal excitability control in health and disease: A neurophysiological comparison of REM sleep and epilepsy. *Progress in Neurobiology, 25*, 141-188.

Elbert, T., Ray, W.J., Kowalik, Z.J., Skinner, J.E., Graf, K.E., and Birbaumer N. (1994). Chaos and Physiology: Deterministic Chaos in Excitable Cell Assemblies. *Physiological Reviews, 74*, 1-47.

Elger, C.E., Widman, G., Andrzejak, R., Arnhold, J., David, P., and Lehnertz, K. (2000). Nonlinear EEG analysis and its potential role in epileptology. *Epilepsia, 41*, Suppl 3:S 34-8.

Elkins, G., White, J., Patel, P., Marcus, J., Perfect, M.M., and Montgomery, G.H. (2006). Hypnosis to manage anxiety and pain associated with colonoscopy for colorectal cancer screening: Case studies and possible benefits. *International Journal of Clinical and Experimental Hypnosis, 54*, 416-31.

Elkins, G., Jensen, M.P., and Patterson, D.R. (2007). Hypnotherapy for the management of chronic pain. *International Journal of Clinical and Experimental Hypnosis, 55*, 275-87.

Ellason, J. W. and Ross, C. A. (1995). Positive and negative symptoms in dissociative identity disorder and schizophrenia: a comparative analysis. *Journal of Nervous and Mental Disease 183*, 236-41.

Ellason, J.W. and Ross, C.A. (1997). Childhood trauma and psychiatric symptoms. *Psychological Reports, 80*, 447-50.

Ellenberger, H.F. (1970). *The Discovery of the Unconscious: The History and Evolution of Dynamic Psychiatry.* New York: Basic.

El-Sherif, Y., Tesoriero, J., Hogan, M.V., and Wieraszko, A. (2003). Melatonin regulates neuronal plasticity in the hippocampus. *Journal of Neuroscience Research, 72,* 454–460.

Epstein, A. W. (1964). Recurrent dreams; their relationship to temporal lobe seizures. *Archives of General Psychiatry, 10,* 49-54.

Esch, T. and Stefano, G.B. (2005). The neurobiology of love. *Activitas Nervosa Superior 49*: 1-18.

Faber, J. and Vladyka, V. (1987). Epileptogenesis and Psychosogenesis, antithesis or synthesis? *Acta Universitatis Carolinae Medica, 34,* 245-312.

Faber, J., Vladyka, V., Dufkova, D., Faltus, F., Jirak, R., Pavlovsky, J., Smidova, E., Zvolsky, P., Zukov, I., Klar, I., Posmurova, M., and Srutova, L. (1996). "Epileptosis"- A syndrome or useless speculation. *Sbornik lekarsky, 97,* 71-95.

Faure, P. and Korn, H. (2001). Is there chaos in the brain? I. Concepts of nonlinear dynamics and methods of investigation. *Comptes rendus de l'Academie des sciences. Serie III,* Sciences de la vie, 324, 773-793.

Faw, B. (1997). Outlining a brain model of mental imaging abilities. *Neuroscience and Biobehavioral Reviews, 21,* 283-288.

Faymonville, M.E., Roediger, L., Del Fiore, G., Delgueldre, C., Phillips, C., Lamy, M., Luxen, A., Maquet, P., and Laureys, S. (2003). Increased cerebral functional connectivity underlying the antinociceptive effects of hypnosis. *Cognitive Brain Research, 17,* 255–262.

Feinberg, I. (1978). Efference copy and corollary discharge: implications for thinking and its disorders. *Schizophrenia Bulletin* 4, 636-40.

Feinberg, I. and Guazzelli, M. (1999). Schizophrenia- a disorder of the corollary discharge systems that integrate the motor systems of thought with the sensory systems of consciousness. *British Journal of Psychiatry 17,* 4196-204.

Feldman, J.B. (2004). The neurobiology of pain, affect and hypnosis. *American Journal of Clinical Hypnosis, 46,* 187-200.

Ferenczi S. (1934). Gedanken über das trauma. *International Zeitschrift für Psychoanalyse, 20,* 5-12.

Fernandez-Duque, D., Grossi, G., Thornton, I.M., and Seville, H.J. (2003). Representation of change: separate electrophysiological markers of attention, awareness, and implicite processing. *Journal of Cognitive Neuroscience, 15,* 491–507.

Fidelman, U. (2005). Visual search and quantum mechanics: A neuropsychological basis of Kant's creative imagination. *Journal of Mind and Behavior, 26,* 23-33.

Fingelkursts, A.A., Fingelkursts, A.A. and Kaplan, Ya.A. (2006). Interictal EEG as a physiological adaptation. Part II. Topographic variability of composition of brain oscillations in interictal EEG. *Clinical Neurophysiology, 117,* 789-802.

Fischer, C. (1954). Dreams and perception: The role of preconscious and primary modes of perception and dream formation. *Journal of the American Psychoanalytic Association ,* 2, 389-445.

Fishbain, D.A., Cutler, R.B., Rosomoff, H.L., and Rosomoff, R.S. (2001). Pain-determined dissociation episodes. *Pain Medicine, 2,* 216-24.

Fisher, R.S., Webber, W.R., Lesser, R.P., Arroyo, S., and Uematsu, S. (1992). High-frequency EEG activity at the start of seizures. *Journal of Clinical Neurophysiology, 9*, 441-448.

Fiss, H. (1986). An empirical foundation for a self psychology of dreaming. *Journal of Mind and Behavior, 7,* 161-192.

Flor-Henry, P. (1969). Psychosis and temporal lobe epilepsy: A controled investigation. *Epilepsia, 10,* 363-395.

Flor-Henry, P. (2003). Lateralized temporal-limbic dysfunction and psychopatology. *Epilepsy and Behaviour, 4,* 578-590.

Foltz, E.L. and Lowell, E.W. (1962). Pain "relief" by frontal cingulumotomy. *Journal of Neurosurgery, 19,* 89-100.

Foltz, E.L. and White, L.E. (1968). The role or rostral cingulumotomy in "pain" relief. *International Journal of Neurology, 6,* 353–373.

Foote, B. and Park, J. (2008). Dissociative identity disorder and schizophrenia: differential diagnosis and theoretical issues. *Current Psychiatry Reports, 10,* 217-222.

Ford, J.M., Mathalon, D.H., Heinks, T., Kalba, S., Faustman, W.O., and Roth, W.T. (2001). Neurophysiological evidence of corollary discharge dysfunction in schizophrenia. *American Journal of Psychiatry, 158,* 2069-71.

Ford, J.M., Gray, M., Faustman, W.O., Heinks, T.H., and Mathalon, D.H. (2005). Reduced gamma-band coherence to distorted feedback during speech when what you say is not what you hear. *International Journal of Psychophysiology, 57,* 143-50.

Ford, J.M., Gray, M., Faustman, W.O., Roach, B.J., and Mathalon, D.H. (2007). Dissecting corollary discharge dysfunction in schizophrenia. *Psychophysiology, 44,* 522-9.

Frances, A. and Spiegel, D. (1987). Chronic pain masks depression, multiple personality disorder. *Hospital and Community Psychiatry, 38,* 933–5.

Frankel, F.H. (1996). Dissociation: The clinical realities. *American Journal of Psychiatry, 153* (Suppl.), 64-70.

Frazer, A., Brown, R., Kocsis, J., Caroff, S., Amsterdam, J., Winokur, A., Sweeney, J., Stokes, P., 1986. Patterns of melatonin rhythms in depression. *Journal of Neural Transmission, Suppl. 21,* 269–290.

Freeman, R. and Schachter, S.C. (1995). Autonomic epilepsy. *Seminars in Neurology, 15,* 158-66.

Freeman, W.J. (1983). The Physiological Basis of Mental Images. *Biological Psychiatry, 18,* 1007-25.

Freeman, W.J. (1991). The physiology of perception. *Scientific American, 264,* 78-85.

Freeman, W.J. (1999). Consciousness, Intentionality, and Causality. *Journal of Consciousness Studies, 6,* 143-172.

Freeman, W.J. (2000). Mesoscopics neurodynamics: From neuron to brain. *Journal of Physiology (Paris), 94,* 303-322.

Freeman, W.J. (2001). Biocomplexity: Adaptive behavior in complex stochastic dynamical systems. *BioSystems, 59,* 109-123.

Frewen, P.A., Pain, C., Dozois, D.J., Lanius, R.A. (2006). Alexithymia in PTSD: psychometric and FMRI studies. *Annals of the New York Academy Sciences, 1071,* 397-400.

Fries, P. (2005). A mechanism for cognitive dynamics: neuronal communication through neuronal coherence. *Trends in Cognitive Sciences, 9*, 474–480.

Fröhlich, H. (1968). Long range coherence and energy storage in biological systems. *International Journal of Quantum Chemistry, 2*, 641-64.

Fröhlich, H. (1970). Long range coherence and the actions of enzymes. *Nature, 228*, 1093.

Fröhlich, H. (1975). The extraordinary dielectric properties of biological materials and the actions of enzymes. *Proceedings of the National Academy of Sciences of the United States of America, 72*, 4211-4215.

Fuchs, E. and Schumacher, M. (1990). Psychosocial stress affects pineal function in the tree shrew (Tupaia belangeri). *Physiology and Behavior, 47*, 713–717.

Funahashi, S. (2001). Neuronal mechanisms of executive control by the prefrontal cortex. *Neuroscience Research, 39*, 147-65.

Gabel, S. (1989). Dreams as a possible reflection of dissociated self-monitoring system. *Journal of Nervous and Mental Disease, 177*, 560-568.

Galin, D. (1974). Implications for psychiatry of left and right cerebral specialization. *Archives of General Psychiatry, 31*, 572-583.

Gawronski, B., Hofmann, W., and Wilbur, C.J. (2006). Are "implicit" attitudes unconscious? *Consciousness and Cognition, 15*, 485-99.

Gazzaniga, M.S. and Sperry, R.W. (1967). Language after section of the cerebral commissures. *Brain, 90*, 131–148.

Gerdin, M.J., Masana, M.I., Rivera-Bermudez, M.A., Hudson, R.L., Earnest, D.J., Gillette. M.U., and Dubocovich, M.L. (2004). Melatonin desensitizes endogenous MT2 melatonin receptors in the rat suprachiasmatic nucleus: relevance for defining the periods of sensitivity of the mammalian circadian clock to melatonin. *FASEB Journal, 18*, 1646–1656.

Gerendai, I. and Halász, B. (2001). Asymmetry of the neuroendocrine system. *News in Physiological Sciences 16*, 92-5.

Ghirardi, G.C., Grassi, R., and Pearle, P. (1990). Relativistic dynamical reduction models: general framework and examples. *Foundations of Physics, 20*, 271-316.

Glaslova, K., Bob, P., Jasova, D., Bratkova, N., Ptacek, R. (2004). Traumatic stress and schizophrenia. *Neurology, Psychiatry and Brain Research, 11*, 205-208.

Ghosh, D., Mohanty, G., and Prabhakar, S. (2001). Ictal deafness- a report of three cases. *Seizure, 10*, 130-133.

Globus, G.C. and Arpaia, J.P. (1994). Psychiatry and the new dynamics. *Biological Psychiatry, 32*, 352-364.

Goddard, G.V., McIntyre, G.C., and Leech, C.K. (1969). A permanent change in brain function resulting from daily electrical stimulation. *Experimental Neurology, 25*, 295-330.

Goebel, R., Khorram-Sefat, D., Muckli, L., Hacker, H., and Singer, W. (1998). The constructive nature of vision: direct evidence from functional magnetic resonance imaging studies of apparent motion and motion imagery. *European Journal of Neuroscience, 10*, 1563–1573.

Goffaux, P., Redmond, W.J., Rainville, P., and Marchand, S. (2007). Descending analgesia- When the spine echoes what the brain expects. *Pain, 130*, 137-143.

Goldberg, T.E. and Weinberger, D.R. (2000). Thought disorder in schizophrenia: A reappraisal of older formulations and an overview of some recent studies. *Cognitive Neuropsychiatry, 5*, 1-19.

Good, M.I. (1993). The Concept of an Organic Dissociative Syndrome: What is the Evidence? *Harvard Review of Psychiatry, 1*, 145-57.

Goodwin, R.D., Fergusson, D.M., and Horwood, L.J. (2005). Childhood abuse and familial violence and the risk of panic attacks and panic disorder in young adulthood. *Psychological Medicíně, , 35*, 881-90.

Goon, Y., Robinson, S., and Lavy, S. (1973). Electroencephalographic changes in schizophrenic patients. *The Israel Annals of Psychiatry and Related Disciplines, 11*, 99-107.

Gorfine, T. and Zisapel, N. (2007). Melatonin and the human hippocampus, a time dependent interplay. *Journal of Pineal Research, 43*, 80-6.

Gottschalk, A. M., Bauer, M. S., and Whybrow, P. C. (1995). Evidence of chaotic mood variation in bipolar disorder. *Archives of General Psychiatry, 52*, 947-959.

Gracely, R.H., Petzke, F., Wolf, J.M., and Clauw, D.J. (2002). Functional magnetic resonance imaging evidence of augmented pain processing in fibromyalgia. *Arthritis and Rheumatism, 46*, 1333– 1343.

Grachev, I.D., Fredrickson, B.E., and Apkarian, A.V. (2000). Abnormal brain chemistry in chronic back pain: an in vivo proton magnetic resonance spectroscopy study. *Pain, 89*, 7-18.

Grachev, I.D., Thomas, P.S., and Ramachandran, T.S. (2002). Decreased levels of N-acetylaspartate in dorsolateral prefrontal cortex in a case of intractable severe sympathetically mediated chronic pain (complex regional pain syndrome, type I). *Brain and Cognition, 49*, 102-13.

Greaves, G.B. (1980). Multiple personality. 165 years after Mary Reynolds. *Journal of Nervous and Mental Disease, 168*, 577–96.

Greenspan, J.D., Lee, R.R., and Selz, F.A. (1999). Pain sensitivity alterations as a function of lesion location in the parasylvian cortex. *Pain, 81*, 273-282.

Groethuysen, V.C., Robinson, D.B., Haylett, C.H., Estes, H.R., and Johnson, A.M. (1957). Depth electrographic recording of a seizure during a structured interview. *Psychosomatic Medicine, 19*, 353-362.

Gruzelier, J.H. (1983). Disparate syndromes in psychosis delineated by direction of electrodermal response lateral asymmetry. In P. Flor-Henry and J. Gruzelier (Eds.), *Laterality and Psychopathology*, pp. 525-538. Amsterdam: Elsevier.

Gruzelier, J.H. and Venables, P.H. (1974). Bimodality and lateral asymmetry of skin conductance orienting activity in schizophrenics: Replication and evidence of lateral asymmetry in patients with depression and disorders of personality. *Biological Psychiatry, 2*, 131-139.

Guralnik, O., Levin, R., and Schmeidler, J. (1999). Dreams of personality disordered subjects. *Journal of Nervous and Mental Disease, 187,* 40-46.

Hagan, S., Hameroff, S.R., and Tuszynski, J.A. (2002). Quantum computation in brain microtubules: Decoherence and biological feasibility. *Physical Review E, 65*, 061901-069101.

Hall, J.M. and Powell, J. (2000). Dissociative experiences described by women survivors of childhood abuse. *Journal of Interpersonal Violence, 15*, 184-204.

Hamada, T., Antle, M.C., Silver, R. (2004). Temporal and spatial expression patterns of canonical clock genes and clock-controlled genes in the suprachiasmatic nucleus. *European Journal of Neuroscience, 19*, 1741-8.

Hameroff, S.R., Penrose, R. (1995). Orchestrated Reduction of Quantum Coherence in Brain Microtubules: A Model for Consciousness. *Neural Network World, 5*, 793.

Hameroff, S.R., and Penrose, R. (1996). Orchestrated reduction of quantum coherence in brain microtubules: A model of consciousness. In S. Hameroff, and A. Kaszniak (Eds). *Toward a science of consciousness* (pp. 507-540). Cambridge: MIT Press.

Hammond, D.C. (2007). Review of the efficacy of clinical hypnosis with headaches and migraines. *International Journal of Clinical and Experimental Hypnosis, 55*, 207-219.

Hardy, S.G.P. and Haigler, H.J. (1985). Prefrontal influences upon the midbrain: a possible route for pain modulation. *Brain Research, 339*, 285-93.

Hartmann, E. (1998). Nightmare after trauma as paradigm for all dreams: A new approach to the nature and functions of dreaming. *Psychiatry, 61*, 223-238.

Haule, J.R. (1984). From Somnambulism to the Archetypes: The French Roots of Jung's Split with Freud. *Psychoanalytic Review, 71*, 636-689.

Havens, L.L. (1966). Pierre Janet. *Journal of Nervous and Mental Disease, 143*, 383-398.

Hazeltine, E., Poldrack, R., and Gabrieli, J.D.E. (2000). Neural activation during response competition. *Journal of Cognitive Neuroscience, 12*, Suppl. 2, 118-129.

Heath, R.G. (1962). Common Characteristic of epilepsy and schizophrenia: Clinical Observation and Depth Electrode Studies. *American Journal of Psychiatry, 118*, 1013-1026.

Heath, R.G. (1975). Brain Function and Behaviour. *Journal of Nervous and Mental Disease, 160*, 159-175.

Heim, C., Newport, D.J., Heit, S., Graham, Y.P., Wilcox, M., Bonsall, R., Miller, A.H., and Nemeroff, C.B. (2000). Pituitary-adrenal and autonomic responses to stress in women after sexual and physical abuse in childhood. *JAMA: the journal of the American Medical Association, 284*, 592-7.

Heisenberg, W. (1958). *Physics and philosophy. The revolution in modern science.* New York: Harper and Row.

Hemby, S.E., Trojanowski, J.Q., and Ginsberg, S.D. (2003). Neuron-specific age-related decreases in dopamine receptor subtype mRNAs. *Journal of Comprehensive Neurology, 456*, 176–183.

Henninger, P. (1992). Conditional handedness: Handedness changes in multiple personality disorder subjects reflect shifts in hemispheric dominance. *Consciousness and Cognition, 1*, 265-287.

Henry, G., Weingartner, H., Murphy, L.D. (1973). Influence of Affective States and Psychoactive Drugs on Verbal Learning and Memory. *American Journal of Psychiatry, 130*, 66-71.

Henry, J.P. (1993). Psychological and physiological responses to stress: the right hemisphere and the hypothalamo-pituitary-adrenal axis, an inquiry into problems of human bonding. *Integretive Physiology and Behavioral Sciences, 28*, 369-87.

Henry, J.P. (1997). Psychological and physiological responses to stress: the right hemisphere and the hypothalamo-pituitary-adrenal axis, an inquiry into problems of human bonding. *Acta Physiologica Scandinavica, 161*, 10-25 (Suppl).

Hersch, J., Yiu-Chung, C., and Smeltzer, D. (2002). Identity shifts in temporal lobe epilepsy. *General Hospital Psychiatry, 24*, 185-187.

Herzog, A.G. (1993). A relationship between particular reproductive endocrine disorders and the laterality of epileptiform discharges in women with epilepsy. *Neurology 43*, 1907–1910

Hilgard, E.R. (1974). Toward a Neodissociation Theory: Multiple Cognitive Controls in Human Functioning. *Perspectives in Biology and Medicine, 17*, 301-316.

Hilgard, E.R. (1986). *Divided Consciousness. Multiple Control in Human Thought and action*. New York: Wiley.

Hilgard, E.R. (1988). Commentary. Professional skepticism about multiple personality. *Journal of Nervous and Mental Disease, 176*, 532.

Hilz, M.J., Dutsch, M., Perrine, K., Nelson, P.K., Rauhut, U., and Devinski, O. (2001). Hemispheric influence on autonomic modulation and baroreflex sensitivity. *Annals of Neurology, 49*, 575-84.

Hines, M., Swan, C., Roberts, R.J., and Varney, N.R. (1995). Characteristics and mechanisms of epilepsy spectrum disorder: An explanatory model. *Applied Neuropsychology, 2*, 1-6.

Hirakawa, N., Tershner, SA, Fields HL, and Manning BH. (2000). Bi-directional changes in affective state elicited by manipulation of medullary pain-modulatory circuitry. *Neuroscience 100*, 861-71.

Hobson, J. A. (1990). Sleep and Dreaming. *Neuroscience, 10*, 371-382.

Hobson, J. A., and McCarley, R. W. (1977). The brain as a dream-state generator: An activation-synthesis hypothesis of the dream process. *American Journal of Psychology, 134*, 1335-1368.

Hobson, J. A., and Pace-Schott, E. F. (2002). The cognitive neuroscience of sleep: Neural systems, consciousness and learning. *Nature Reviews Neuroscience, 3*, 679-693.

Hofbauer, R.K., Rainville, P., Duncan, G.H., and Bushnell, C. (2001). Cortical representation of the sensory dimension of pain. *Journal of Neurophysiology, 86*, 402-411.

Hoffman, R.E., Kirstein, L., Stopek, S., and Cicchetti, D.V. (1982). Apprehending schizophrenic dicourse: A structural analysis of the listener's task. *Brain and Language, 15*, 207-233.

Hogan, M.V., El-Sherif, Y., and Wieraszko, A. (2001). The modulation of neuronal activity by melatonin: in vitro studies on mouse hippocampal slices. *Journal of Pineal Research, 30*, 87–96.

Holloway, F.A. (1978). State Dependent Learning and Time of Day. *In Drug Discrimination and State Dependent Learning*, Eds. Ho, B.T., Richards, D.V., Chute, D.L., London: Academic Press.

Horowitz, M., Wilner, M., and Alvarez, W. (1979). Impact of Event Scale: A Measure of Subjective Stress. *Psychosomatic Medicine, 41*, 209-218.

Horowitz, M.J. (1986). *Stress response syndromes*, 2nd ed. Northvale, NJ: Jason Aronson.

Hotchkiss, A.P. and Harvey, P.D. (1990). Effect of distraction on communication failures in schizophrenic patients. *Clinical Research Reports, 147*, 513–515.

Huang, C.M. and White, L.E. Jr. (1989). High-frequency components in epileptiform EEG. *Journal of Neuroscience Methods, 30*, 197-201.

Huber, M.T., Braun, H.A., and Krieg, J.C. (1999). Consequences of deterministic and random dynamics for the course of affective disorders. *Biological Psychiatry, 46*, 256-262.

Hugdahl, K. (2001). *Psychophysiology, The Mind-Body Perspective*. Cambridge: Harvard University Press.

Huston, P., Skehow, J., and Erickson, M. (1934). A Study of Hypnotically Induced Complexes by Means of the Louria Technique. *Journal of General Psychology, 11*, 65-97.

Iezzi, T., Archibald, Y., Barnett, P., Klinck, A., and Duckwork M. (1999). Neurocognitive performance and emotional status in chronic pain patients. *Journal of Behavioral Medicine, 22*, 205-16.

Indic, P., Schwartz, W.J., Herzog, E.D., Foley, N.C., and Antle, M.C. (2007). Modeling the behavior of coupled cellular circadian oscillators in the suprachiasmatic nucleus. *Journal of Biological Rhythms, 22*, 211-9.

Inoue, M. and Nakamoto, K. (1994). Dynamics of Cognitive Interpretations of a Necker Cube in a Chaos Neural Network. *Progress of Theoretical Physics, 92*, 501-508.

International Association for the Study of Pain Task Force on Taxonomy (1994). Classification of chronic pain: Descriptions of chronic pain syndromes and definitions of pain terms. Seattle: IASP Press.

Isaacs, A., Daintith, J., and Martin, E. (2003). *Oxford Dictionary of Science*. New York: Oxford University Press.

Isenberg, N., Silbersweig, D., Engelien, A., Emmerich, S., Malavade, K., Beattie, B., and Leon, A.C. (1999). Linguistic threat activates the human amygdala. *Proceedings of the National Academy of Sciences of the United States of America 96*, 10456-10459.

Ito, Y., Teicher, M., Gold, C., Harper, D., Magnus, E., and Gelbard, H. (1993). Increased prevalence of electrophysiological abnormalities in children with psychological, physical and sexual abuse. *Journal of Neuropsychiatry and Clinical Neuroscience, 5*, 401-408.

Ito, Y., Teicher, M.H., Glod, C.A., and Ackerman, E. (1998). Preliminary evidence for aberrant cortical development in abused children: a quantitative EEG study. *Journal of Neuropsychiatry and Clinical Neuroscience, 10*, 298-307.

Jacobs, W.J. and Nadel, L. (1985). Stress induced recovery of fears and phobias. *Psychological Review, 92*, 512-531.

Jacobs, W.J. and Nadel L. (1999). The first panic attack: a neurobiological theory. Canadian *Journal of Experimental Psychology, 53*, 92-107.

Jampala, V., Atre-Vaidya, N., and Taylor, M.A. (1992). A profile of psychomotor symptoms (POPS) in psychiatric patients. *Neuropsychiatry, Neuropsychology and Behavioural Neurology, 5*, 15-19.

Janet, P. (1886). Les actes inconscients et le dédoublement de la personnalité pendant le somnambulisme provoqué. *Revue Philosphique, 22*, II, 577-592.

Janet, P. (1890). *L'Automatisme Psychologique*. Paris: Felix Alcan.

Jeans, R.F. (1976). The three faces of Evelyn: A case report. I. An independently validated case of multiple personalities. *Journal of Abnormal Psychology, 85*, 249-255.

Jensen, F.E. and Baram, T.Z. (2000). Developmental seizures induced by common early-life insults: short- and long-term effects on seizure susceptibility. *Mental retardation and developmental disabilities research reviews, 6*, 253-7.

Jensen, M.P. and Patterson, D.R. (2005). Control conditions in hypnotic-analgesia clinical trials: challenges and recommendations. *International Journal of Clinical and Experimental Hypnosis, 53*, 170-97.

Jensen, M.P., McArthur, K.D., Barber, J., Hanley, M.A., Engel, J.M., Romano, J.M., Cardenas, D.D., Kraft, G.H., Hoffman, A.J., and Patterson, D.R. (2006). Satisfaction with, and the beneficial side effects of, hypnotic analgesia. *International Journal of Clinical and Experimental Hypnosis, 54*, 432-47.

Jiang, Z.G., Nelson, C.S., and Allen, C.N. (1995). Melatonin activates an outward current and inhibits Ih in rat suprachiasmatic nucleus neurons. *Brain Research, 687*, 125–132.

Jindal, R.D. and Thase, M.E. (2004). Treatment of insomnia associated with clinical depression. *Sleep Medicine Reviews 8*, 19–30.

Jobe, P.C., Dailey, J.W., and Wernicke, J.F. (1999). A Noradrenergic and Serotoninergic Hypothesis of the Linkage between Epilepsy and Affective Disorders. *Critical Reviews in Neurobiology, 13*, 317-356.

John, E.R. (2002). The neurophysics of consciousness. *Brain Research Reviews, 39*, 1-28.

Jonides, J., Smith, E.E., Marshuetz, C., Koeppe, R.A., and Reuter-Lorenz, P.A. (1998). Inhibition of verbal working memory revealed by brain activation. *Proceedings of the National Academy of Sciences of the United States of America, 95*, 8410-13.

Jung, C.G. (1907). On psychophysical relations of the associative experiment. *Journal of Abnormal Psychology, 1*, 247-255.

Jung, C.G. (1909). The Psychology of Dementia Praecox. New York: *Journal of Nervous and Mental Disease Publishing Company*, (also in Collected Works of C. G. Jung 3).

Jung, C.G. (1968). *Analytical Psychology: Its Theory and Practice*. London: Routledge and Kegan Paul,.

Jung, C.G. (1972). The transcendent function. In *Collected Works* of C. G. Jung. 8. Princeton: University Press (p. 67-91).

Jung, C. G. (1972a). On the Nature of the Psyche. The structure and dynamics of the psyche. In: *Collected Works* of C.G. Jung 8, Princeton: Princeton University Press.

Jung, C. G. (1972b). Psychological factors determining human behaviour. The structure and dynamics of the psyche. In: *Collected Works* of C.G. Jung 8. Princeton: Princeton University Press.

Jung, C. G. (1972c). A Review of the Complex Theory. The structure and dynamics of the psyche. In: *Collected Works* of C.G. Jung 8. Princeton: Princeton University Press.

Jung, C. G. (1973). Collected Works of C. G. Jung 2. Princeton: Princeton University Press.

Jung, C.G. (1989). Mysterium coniunctionis. *Collected works* of C.G. Jung XIV. Princeton: Princeton University Press.

Jung, C.G. (1972). Aion. *Collected works* of C.G. Jung IX. Princeton: Princeton University Press.

Kaczmarek, L. K., and Babloyantz, A. (1977). Spatiotemporal patterns in epileptic seizures. *Biological Cybernetics, 26*, 199-208.

Kahn, D., and Hobson, J.A. (1993). Self-Organization Theory of Dreaming. *Dreaming, 3*, 151-178.

Kahn, D., Pace-Schott, E. F., and Hobson, J. A. (1997). Consciousness in waking and dreaming: The roles of neuronal oscillation and neuromodulation in determining similarities and differences. *Neuroscience, 78*, 13-38.

Kahn, D., Krippner, S., and Combs, A. (2000). Dreaming and the self-organizing brain. *Journal of Consciousness Studies, 7*, 4-11.

Kahn, D., Krippner, S., and Combs, A. (2002). Dreaming as a Function of Chaos-Like Stochastic Processes in the Self-Organizing Brain. *Nonlinear Dynamics, Psychology and Life Sciences, 6*, 311-322.

Kalsbeek, A., Palm, I.F., La Fleur, S.E., Scheer, F.A., Perreau-Lenz, S., Ruiter, M., Kreier, F., Cailotto, C., and Buijs, R.M. (2006). SCN outputs and the hypothalamic balance of life. *Journal of Biological Rhythms, 21*, 458-69.

Kanner, A. M. (2000). Psychosis of Epilepsy: A Neurologist's Perspective. *Epilepsy and Behaviour, 1*, 219-227.

Kanner, A. M. (2001). The Behavioural Aspects of Epilepsy: An Overview of Controversial Issues, *Epilepsy and Behaviour, 2*, 8-12.

Kanner, A.M. and Balabanov, A. (2002). Depression and Epilepsy. How closely related are they? *Neurology, 58*, 827-839.

Kantz, H. and Schreiber, T. (1997). *Nonlinear time series analysis*. Cambridge: Cambridge University Press.

Kanwisher, N. (2001). Neural events and perceptual awareness. *Cognition, 79*, 89-113.

Kaplan, H. I. and Sadock, B.J. (1991). *Comprehensive Glossary of Psychiatry and Psychology*. Baltimore: Williams and Wilkins.

Kenardy, J., Smith, A., Spence, S.H., Lilley, P.R., Newcombe, P., Dob, R., and Robinson S. (2007). Dissociation in children's trauma narratives: an exploratory investigation. *Journal of Anxiety Disorders, 21*, 456-66.

Kihlstrom, J.F. (1987). The Cognitive Unconscious. *Science, 237*, 1445-1452.

Kihlstrom, J.F. (2004). Availability, accessibility, and subliminal perception. *Consciousness and Cognition, 13*, 92-100.

Kihlstrom, J.F. (2005). Dissociative disorders. *Annual Review of Clinical Psychology 1*, 227-253.

King, C. (1991). Fractal and chaotic dynamics in nervous system. *Progress in Neurobiology, 36*, 279-308.

King, C. (1997). Quantum mechanics, chaos and the conscious brain. *Journal of Mind and Behavior, 18*, 155-170.

Kirsch, I. and Lynn, S. J. (1998). Dissociation theories of hypnosis. *Psychological Bulletin, 123*, 100-115.

Knox, J.M. (2001). Memories, fantasies, archetypes: an exploration of some connections between cognitive science and analytical psychology. *Journal of Analytical Psychology, 46*, 613–633.

Kooiman, C.G., van Rees Vellinga, S., Spinhoven, P., Draijer, N., Trijsburg, R.W., and Rooijmans, H.G. (2004). Childhood adversities as risk factors for alexithymia and other aspects of affect dysregulation in adulthood. *Psychotherapy Psychosomatics, 73*, 107-16.

Korn, H. and Faure, P. (2003). Is there chaos in the brain? II. Experimental evidence and related models. *Comptes Rendus Biologies, 326,* 787-840.

Kosslyn, S.M., Thompson, W.L., Constantini-Ferrando, M.F., Alpert, N.M., and Spiegel, D. (2000). Hypnotic visual illusion alters color processing in the brain. *American Journal of Psychiatry, 157,* 1279-1284.

Kraus, J.E. (2000). Sensitization phenomena in psychiatric illness: Lessons from the kindling model. *Journal of Neuropsychiatry and Clinical Neurosciences, 12,* 328-342.

Krishnamoortthy, E.S., Trimble, M.R., Sander, J.W.A.S., Kanner, and Andres. M. (2002). Forced normalization at the interface between epilepsy and psychiatry. *Epilepsy and Behaviour*, 3, 303-308.

Kruger, C. and Mace, C.J. (2002). Psychometric validation of the State Scale of Dissociation (SSD). *Psychology and Psychotherapy, 75,* 33-51.

Kuramoto,Y. (1984). *Chemical oscillations, waves and turbulence.* New York: Dover Publication.

Kuttner, F. and Rosenblum, B. (2006). The only objective evidence for consciousness. *Journal of Mind and Behavior, 27,* 43-56.

Kuyk, J., Spinhoven, P., Van Emde Boas, W., and Van Dyck, R. (1999). Dissociation in Temporal Lobe Epilepsy and Pseudo-Epileptic Seizure Patients. *Journal of Nervous and Mental Disease , 187,* 713-720.

Kuyken, W. and Brewin, C.R. (1996). Autobiographical memory functioning in depression and reports of early abuse. *Journal of Abnormal Psychology, 1*04, 585-591.

La Bar, K.S., Gatenby, J.C., Gore, J.C., Le Doux, J.E., and Phelps, E.A. (1998). Human amygdala activation during conditioned fear acquisition and extinction: A mixed-trial fMRI study. *Neuron, 20,* 937-945.

Lachaux, J.P., Rodriguez, E., Martinerie, J., and Varela, F.J. (1999). Measuring phase synchrony in brain signals. *Human Brain Mapping, 8,* 194–208.

Lambie, J. A. and Marcel, A.J. (2002). Consciousness and the varieties of emotion experience: a theoretical framework. *Psychological Review, 109,* 219-59.

Lambie, J. A. and Marcel, A.J. (2004). How many selves in emotion experience? Reply to Dalgleish and Power (2004). *Psychological Review, 111,* 820-6.

Landolt, H. (1953). Some clinical electroencephalographical correlations in epileptic psychosis (twilight states). *Electroencephalography and Clinical Neurophysiology, 5,* 121.

Larmore, K., Ludwig, A.M., and Cain, R.L. (1977). Multiple personality: an objective case study. British Journal of Psychiatry, 31, 3540.

Larson, J., Jessen, R.E., Uz, T., Arslan, A.D., Kurtuncu, M., Imbesi, M., and Manev, H. (2006). Impaired hippocampal long-term potentiation in melatonin MT2 receptor-deficient mice. *Neuroscience Letters, 393,* 23-6.

Laudon, M., Hyde, J.F., and Ben-Jonathan, N. (1989). Ontogeny of prolactin releasing and inhibiting activities in the posterior pituitary of male rats. *Neuroendocrinology, 50,* 644–649.

Laurikainen, K.V. (1988). *Beyond the atom: The philosophical thought of Wolfgang Pauli.* Berlin: SpringerVerlag.

Le Page, K.E., Schafer, D. V., and Miller A. (1992). Alternating unilateral lachrymation. *American Journal of Clinical Hypnosis, 34*, 255-260.

LeDoux, J.E. (1992). Brain mechanisms of emotion and emotional learning. *Current Opinion in Neurobiology, 2*, 191-198.

LeDoux, J. E. (1993). Emotional memory systems in the brain. *Behavioural Brain Research, 58*, 69-79.

LeDoux, J. E. (1994). Emotion, memory and the brain. *Scientific American, 270*, 50-57.

Lee, K.H., Williams, L.M., Breakspear, M., and Gordon, E. (2003). Synchronous gamma activity: a review and contribution to an integrative neuroscience model of schizophrenia. *Brain Research Reviews, 41*, 57-78.

Lee, J.L, Everitt, B.J., and Thomas, K.L. (2004). Independent Cellular Processes for Hippocampal Memory Consolidation and Reconsolidation. *Science*, 304, 839-43.

Leff, J. (1994). Stress reduction in the social environment of schizophrenic patients. *Acta Psychiatrica Scandinavica, 384*, Suppl.,133–139.

Lehnertz, K. (1999). Non-linear time series analysis of intracranial EEG recordings in patiens with epilepsy- an overview. *International Journal of Psychophysiology, 34*, 45-52.

Leroy, F., Pezard, L., Nandrino, J.L., and Beaune D. (2005). Dynamical quantification of schizophrenic speech. *Psychiatry Research, 133*, 159-71.

Lesley, J. (2006). Awareness is relative: dissociation as the organisation of meaning. *Consciousness and Cognition, 15*, 593-604.

Leung, H.C., Skudlarski, P., Gatenby, J.C., Peterson, B.S., and Gore, J.C. (2000). An event-related functional MRI study of the Stroop color word interference task. *Cerebral Cortex, 10*, 552-60.

Levinson, B.W. (1967). States of awareness during general anestezia. In J. Lassner (Ed.) Hypnosis and psychosomatic medicine. *Proceedings of the International Congres for Hypnosis and Psychosomatic Medicine*, (pp. 200-207). New York: Springer.

Levitan, H. (1980). The dream in traumatic states. In J.M. Natterson (Ed.), *The Dream in Clinical Practice*. New York: Jason Aronson.

Li, D. and Spiegel, D. (1992). A Neural Network Model of Dissociative Disorders. *Psychiatric Annals, 22*, 144-47.

Libet, B. (1998). Do the models offer testable proposals of brain functions for conscious experience. In H.H. Jasper, L. Descarries, V.C. Costelucci, and S. Rossignol (Eds.), *Advances in neurology: Consciousness at the frontiers of neuroscience* (pp. 213–217). Philadelphia: Lippincott-Raven.

Libet, B., Wright, E.W. Jr, Einstein, B., and Pearl D.K. (1979). Subjective Refferal of the Timing for a Conscious Sensory Experience. *Brain, 102*, 193-224.

Liddell, B.J., Williams, L.M., Rathjen, J., Shevrin, H., and Gordon, E. (2004). A temporal dissociation of subliminal versus supraliminal fear perception: an event-related potential study. *Journal of Cognitive Neuroscience, 16*, 479-86.

Livengood, J.M., Zouny, C.M., and Parris, C.V. (1994). Implications of multiple personality disorder for treatment of chronic pain. *Pain Digest, 4*, 191 4.

Lorenz, J., Cross, D., Minoshima, S., Morrow, T., Paulson, P., and Casey, K. (2002). A unique representation of heat allodynia in the human brain. *Neuron, 35*, 383-93.

Lorenz, J., Minoshima, S., and Casey, K.L. (2003). Keeping pain out of mind. *Brain, 126*, 1079-1091.

Loscher, W., Jackel, R., Czucvar, J. (1986). Is amygdala kindling in rats a model for drug-resistant partial epilepsy? *Experimental Neurology, 93*, 211-226.

Luck, S.J. and Girelli, M. (1998). Electrophysiological approaches to the study of selective attention in the human brain. In *The attentive brain*. Ed. R. Parasuraman. Cambridge: MIT Press , 71–94.

Luoto, S., Taimela, S., Hurri, H., and Alaranta, H. (1999). Mechanisms explaining the association between low back trouble and deficits in information processing. A controlled study with follow-up. *Spine, 24*, 255 61.

Lutzenberger, W., Birbaumer, N., Flor, H., Rockstroh, B., and Elbert, T. (1992). Dimensional Analysis of the Human EEG and Inteligence. *Neuroscience Letters, 143*, 10-14.

Lynn, S.J., Maré, C., Kvaal, S., Segal, D., and Sivec, H. (1994). The Hidden Observer, Hypnotic dreams, and Age regression: Clinical Implications. *American Journal of Clinical Hypnosis, 37*,130-142.

Lynn, S. J., Kirsch, I., Barabasz, A., Cardena, E., and Patterson, D. (2000). Hypnosis as an empirically supported clinical intervention: The state of the evidence and a look to the future. *International Journal of Clinical and Experimental Hypnosis, 48*, 235-255.

Maaranen, P., Tanskanen, A., Honkalampi, K., Haatainen, K., Hintikka, J., and Viinamaki, H. (2005). Factors associated with pathological dissociation in the general population. Australian and New Zealand *Journal of Psychiatry, 39*, 387-94.

MacDonald, A.W., Cohen, J.D., Stenger, V.A., and Carter, C.S. (2000). Dissociating the role of the dorsolateral prefrontal and anterior cingulate cortex in cognitive control. *Science, 288*, 1835-8.

Mace, C.J. (1992). Hysterical conversion I: A history. *British Journal of Psychiatry, 161*, 369-77.

Mace, C.J. (1993). Epilepsy and schizophrenia. *British Journal of Psychiatry, 163*, 439-445.

Mace, C.J. and Trimble, M.R. (1991). Psychosis following temporal lobe epilepsy: a report of six cases. *Journal of Neurology, Neurosurgery and Psychiatry, 54*, 639-644.

Mangina, C.A. and Beuzeron-Mangina, J.H. (1996). Direct electrical stimulation of specific human brain structures and bilateral electrodermal activity. *International Journal of Psychophysiology, 22*, 1-8.

Manschreck, T.C., Maher, B.A, Rucklos, M.E., and White, M.T. (1979). The predictability of thought disordered speech in schizophrenic patients. *British Journal of Psychiatry, 134*, 595–601.

Mansfield, V., and Spiegelman, J. M. (1989). Quantum mechanics and Jungian psychology: Building a bridge. *Journal of Analytical Psychology, 34*, 3-31.

Mansfield, V., and Spiegelman, J. M. (1991). The opposites in quantum mechanics and Jungian psychology Part I: Theoretical foundations. *Journal of Analytical Psychology, 36*, 267-287.

Marshall, I.N. (1989). Consciousness and Bose-Einstein condensates. *New Ideas in Psychology, 7*, 73-83.

Marcel, A.J. (1983). Conscious and Unconscious Perception: An Approach to the Relations Between Phenomenal Experience and Perceptual Processes. *Cognitive Psychology, 15*, 238-300.

Maroun, M. and Richter-Levin, G. (2003). Exposure to acute stress blocks the induction of long-term potentiation of the amygdala-prefrontal cortex pathway in vivo. *Journal of Neuroscience, 23*, 4406-09.

Marsh, L. and Rao, V. (2002). Psychiatric complications in patients with epilepsy: a review. *Epilepsy Research, 49*, 11-33.

Marmer, S. S. (1980a). The dream in dissociative states. In J.M. Natterson (Ed.), *The Dream in Clinical Practice*. New York: Jason Aronson.

Marmer, S.S. (1980b). Psychoanalysis of multiple personality. *International Journal of Psycho-Analysis, 61*, 439-459.

Mason, R. and Rusak, B. (1990). Neurophysiological responses to melatonin in the SCN of short-day sensitive and refractory hamsters. *Brain Research, 533*, 15–19.

Mason, J.W., Wang, S., Yehuda, R., Riney, S., Charney, D.S., and Southwick, S.M. (2001). Psychogenic lowering of urinary cortisol levels linked to increased emotional numbing and a shame-depressive syndrome in combat-related posttraumatic stress disorder. *Psychosomatic Medicine, 63*, 387-401.

Mc Clelland, J.L., Rumelhart, D.E., and the PDP research group: *Parallel Distributed Processing I,II*. Cambridge: MIT Press 1986.

McDowell, M. J. (2001). The three gorillas: an archetype orders a dynamic system. *Journal of Analytical Psychology, 46*, 637-654.

McFadden, I.J. and Woitalla, V.F. (1993). Differing reports of pain perception by different personalities in a patient with chronic pain and multiple personality disorder. *Pain, 55*, 37982.

McFadden, I.J. (1992). Multiple personality disorder becoming manifest after persistence of a chronic pain syndrome. *Clinical Journal of Pain, 8*, 63.

McGrath, J. (1991). Ordering thoughts on thought disorder. *British Journal of Psychiatry, 158*, 307-316.

McNamara, M.E., Fogel, B.S. (1990). Anticonvulsant-responsive panic attacks with temporal lobe EEG abnormalities. *Journal of Neuropsychiatry and Clinical Neuroscience, 2*, 193–196.

Meares, R. (1999). The Contribution of Hughlings Jackson to an Understanding of Dissociation. *American Journal of Psychiatry, 156*, 1850-1855.

Meduna, L. (1935). Versuche über die biologische Beeinflussung des Ablaufes der Schizophrenie. In: Campher- und Cardiazolkräfe. *Zeitschrift für Neurologie und Psychiatrie, 152*, 235-262.

Meduna, L. (1934). Über experimentelle Campherepilepsie. *Archiv für Psychiatrie, 102*, 333-339.

Medvedev, A.V. (2001). Temporal binding at gamma frequencies in the brain: paving the way to epilepsy? *Australasian Physical and Engineering Sciences in Medicine, 24*, 37-48.

Medvedev, A.V. (2002). Epileptiform spikes desynchronize and diminish fast (gamma) activity of the brain. An "antibinding" mechanism? *Brain Research Bulletin, 58*, 115-128.

Melancon, G. and Joanette, Y. (2000). Chaos, Brain and Cognition: Toward a Nonlinear Order? *Brain and Cognition, 42*, 33-36.

Melzack, R. (1999). From the gate to neuromatrix. *Pain, 6* (Suppl.), 121-126.

Melzack, R. (2001). Pain and the neuromatrix in the brain. *Journal of Dental Education, 65*, 1378-82.

Melzack, R. and Casey, K.L. (1968). Sensory, motivational and central control mechanisms of pain: A new conceptual model. In D. Kanshelo (ed.) *The Skin Senses*, (pp. 423-439). Springfield: Charles C. Thomas.

Merckelbach, H., Rassin, E., and Muris, P. (2000). Dissociation, schizotypy, and fantasy proneness in undergraduate students. *Journal of Nervous and Mental Disease, 88*, 428-31.

Merikle, P. M., Smilek, D., and Eastwood, J. D. (2001). Perception without awareness: perspectives from cognitive psychology. *Cognition, 79*, 115-134.

Merskey, H. (1992). The manufacture of personalities. The production of multiple personality disorders. *British Journal of Psychiatry, 160*, 327-40.

Mesulam, M.M. (1981). Dissociative states with abnormal temporal lobe EEG. *Archives of Neurology, 38*, 176-181.

Mesulam, M.M. (1999). Neural substrates of behaviour: The effects of focal brain lesions upon mental states. In Nicholi, A.M. (ed.), *The Harvard Guide to Psychiatry*. The Belknap Press of Harvard University Press, Cambridge.

Metzinger, T. (2000). The subjectivity of subjective experience: A representationalist analysis of the first person perspective. In T. Metzinger (Ed.), *Neural Correlates of Consciousness: Empirical and Conceptual Questions* (pp. 285-306). Cambridge: MIT Press.

Meyer, U., Kruhoffer, M., Flugge, G., and Fuchs, E. (1998). Cloning of glucocorticoid receptor and mineralocorticoid receptor cDNA and gene expression in the central nervous system of the tree shrew (Tupaia belangeri). *Molecular Brain Research, 55*, 243–253.

Meyer-Lindenberg, A., Zeman, U., Hajak, G., Cohen, L., and Berman, K.F. (2002). Transitions between dynamical states of differing stability in the human brain. *Proceedings of the National Academy of Sciences of the United States of America, 99*, 10948-10953.

Milin, J., Demajo, M., and Todorovic, V., 1996. Rat pinealocyte reactive response to a long-term stress inducement. *Neuroscience 73*, 845–854.

Miller RJ (1992). Is there a neural basis for borderline splitting? *Comprehensive Psychiatry 33*, 92-104.

Mizuno, K. and Giese, K.P. (2005). Hippocampus-dependent memory formation: do memory type-specific mechanisms exist? *Journal of Pharmacological Sciences, 98*, 191-7.

Mölle, M., Marshall, L., Lutzenberger, W., Pietrowsky, R., Fehm, H.L. and Born J. (1996). Enhanced Dynamic Complexity in the Human EEG during Creative Thinking. *Neuroscience Letters, 208*, 61-64.

Monroe, R. R. (1978). The Episodic Psychoses of Vincent van Gogh. *Journal of Nervous and Mental Disease, 166*, 480-488.

Monroe, R. R. (1982). Limbic Ictus and Atypical Psychoses. *Journal of Nervous and Mental Disease, 170*, 711-716.

Montgomery, G. H., DuHamel, K. N., and Redd, W. H. (2000). A meta-analysis of hypnotically induced analgesia: how effective is hypnosis? *International Journal of Clinical and Experimental Hypnosis, 48*, 138-153.

Morris, J.S., Ohman, A., and Dolan, R.J. (1999). A subcortical pathway to the right amygdala mediating "unseen" fear. *Proceedings of the National Academy of Sciences of the United States of America 96*, 1680-1685.

Morrison, A.P., Frame, L., and Larkin, W. (2003). Relationships between trauma and psychosis: a review and integration. *British Journal of Clinical Psychology, 42*, 331-53.

Mossner, R., Daniel, S., Albert, D., Heils, A., Okladnova, O., Schmitt, A., and Lesch, K.P. (2000). Serotonin transporter function is modulated by brain derived neurotrophic factor (BDNF) but not nerve growth factor (NGF). *Neurochemistry International, 36*, 197–202.

Musshoff, U., Riewenherm, D., Berger, E., Fauteck, J.D., and Speckmann, E.J. (2002). Melatonin receptors in rat hippocampus: molecular and functional investigations. *Hippocampus, 12*, 165–173.

Nadel, L. (1994). Hippocampus, space, and relations. *Behavioural and Brain Sciences, 17*, 490-491.

Nadel, L. and Jacobs, W.J. (1998). Traumatic memory is special. *Current Directions in Psychological Science, 7*, 154-157.

Narita, M., Aoki, K., Takagi, M., Yajima, Y., and Suzuki, T. (2003). Implication of brain derived neurotrophic factor in the release of dopamine and dopamine-related behaviors induced by amphetamine. *Neuroscience, 119*, 767–775.

Nasrallah, H.A. (1985). The unintegrated right cerebral hemispheric consciousness as alien intruder: A possible mechanism for schneiderian delusions in schizophrenia. *Comprehensive Psychiatry, 26*, 273-282.

Natsoulas, T. (2006). The case for intrinsic theory: XII. Inner awareness conceived of as a modal character of conscious experiences. *Journal of Mind and Behavior, 27*, 183-213.

Nemiah, J.C. (1981). Dissociative Disorders. In A.M Freeman and H.I. Kaplan. (Ed.), *Comprehensive Textbook of Psychiatry*. Third edition. Williams and Wilkins, Baltimore.

Nijenhuis, E.R.S. (2000). Somatoform dissociation: major symptoms of dissociative disorders. *Journal of Trauma and Dissociation, 1*, 7-32.

Nijenhuis, E.R.S., Spinhoven, Ph., Van Dyck, R., Van Der Hart O. and Vanderlinden, J. (1996). The development and psychometric characteristics of the somatoform dissociation questionnaire (SDQ- 20). *Journal of Nervous and Mental Disease, 184*, 688-694.

Nijenhuis, E. R. S., Spinhoven, P., Vanderlinden, J., van Dyck, R., van der Hart, O. (1998). Somatoform dissociative symptoms as related to animal defensive reactions to predatory imminence and injury. *Journal of Abnormal Psychology, 107*, 63–73.

Nijenhuis, E.R., van der Hart, O., Kruger, K., Steele, K. (2004). Somatoform dissociation, reported abuse and animal defence-like reactions. *Australian and New Zealand Journal of Psychiatry, 8*, 678-86.

Nogrady, H., McConkey, K.M., Laurence, J.R., and Perry, C. (1983). Dissociation, Duality and Demand Characteristics in Hypnosis. *Journal of Abnormal Psychology, 90*, 334-344.

Norman, R. M. and Malla, A. K. (1993). Stressful life events and schizophrenia. I: A review of the research. *British Journal of Psychiatry, 162*, 161–166.

O'Brien, M. (1985). The diagnosis of multiple personality syndromes: overt, covert, and latent. *Comprehensive Therapy, 11*, 59-66.

Ochsner, K.N., Kosslyn, S.M., Cosgrove, G.R., Cassem, E.H., Price, B.H., Nierenberg, A.A., and Rauch, S.L. (2001). Deficits in visual cognition and attention following bilateral anterior cingulotomy. *Neuropsychologia, 39*, 219-30.

Olypher, A.V., Klement, D., Fenton, A.A., 2006. Cognitive disorganization in hippocampus: A physiological model of the disorganization in psychosis. *Journal of Neuroscience, 26*, 158-168.

Orbach, I., Mikulincer, M., King, R., Cohen, D., and Stein, D. (1997). Thresholds and tolerance of physical pain in suicidal and nonsuicidal adolescents. *Journal of Consulting and Clinical Psychology, 65*, 646-652.

Orr, S.P. and Roth, W.T. (2000). Psychophysiological assessment: clinical applications for PTSD. *Journal of Affective Disorders, 61*, 225-240.

Overton, D.A. (1978). Major Theories of State Dependent Learning. In Drug Discrimination and State Dependent Learning, Eds. Ho, B.T., Richards, D.V., Chute, D.L., Academic Press, London.

Ozcan, M., Yilmaz, B., and Carpenter, D.O. (2006). Effects of melatonin on synaptic transmission and long-term potentiation in two areas of mouse hippocampus. *Brain Research, 1111*, 90-94.

Pacchierotti, C., Iapichino, S., Bossini, L., Pieraccini, F., and Castrogiovanni, P. (2001). Melatonin in psychiatric disorders: a review on the melatonin involvement in psychiatry. *Frontiers in Neuroendocrinology, 22*, 18-32.

Packard, R.C. and Brown, F. (1986). Multiple headaches in a case of multiple personality disorder. *Headache, 26*, 99 102.

Pakalnis, A., Drake, M.E., Kuruvilla, J., and Blake, J.K. (1988). Forced normalization. *Archives of Neurology, 45*, 139.

Panksepp, J. (2003). Feeling the pain of social loss. *Science, 302*, 237-239.

Patel, T., Brewin, C.R., Wheatley, J., Wells, A., Fisher, P., and Myers, S. (2007). Intrusive images and memories in major depression. *Behaviour Research and Therapy, 45*, 2573-80.

Patterson, D. R. and Jensen, M. P. (2003). Hypnosis and clinical pain. *Psychological Bulletin, 129*, 495-521.

Patterson, D.R., Wiechman, S.A., Jensen, M., and Sharar, S.R. (2006). Hypnosis delivered through immersive virtual reality for burn pain: A clinical case series. *International Journal of Clinical and Experimental Hypnosis, 54*, 130-42.

Paulsen, J.S., Romero, R., Chan, A., Davis, A.V., Heaton, R.K., and Jeste, D.V. (1996). Impairment of the semantic network in schizophrenia. *Psychiatry Research, 63*, 109–121.

Paulus, M.P. and Braff, D.L. (2003). Chaos and Schizophrenia: Does the method fit the madness? *Biological Psychiatry, 53*, 3-11.

Paus, T. (2001). Primate anterior cingulated cortex: where motor control, drive and cognition interface. *Nature Reviews Neuroscience, 2*, 417-424.

Payne, J.D., Jackson, E.D., Ryan, L., Hoscheidt, S., Jacobs, J.W., and Nadel, L. (2006). The impact of stress on neutral and emotional aspects of episodic memory. *Memory, 14*, 1-16.

Pearce, S., Isherwood, S., Hrouda, D., Richardson, P., Erskine, A. and Skinner, J. (1990). Memory and pain; tests of mood congruity and state dependent learning in experimentally induced and clinical pain. *Pain, 43*, 187–193.

Pediaditakis, N. (1992). Deterministic non-linear chaos in brain function and borderline psychopathological phenomena. *Medical Hypotheses, 39*, 67-72.

Peled, A. (1999). Multiple constraint organization in the brain: a theory for schizophrenia. *Brain Research Bulletin, 49*, 245-50.

Penrose, R. (1989). *The Emperor's new mind: Concerning computers, minds, and the laws of physics*. Oxford: Oxford University Press.

Penrose, R. (1994). *Shadows of the mind: An approach to the missing science of consciousness*. Oxford: Oxford University Press.

Penrose, R. (1997). *The large the small and the human mind*. Cambridge: The Press Syndicate of the University of Cambridge.

Penrose, R. (2001). Consciousness, the brain, and spacetime geometry: An addendum. *Annals of the New York Academy of Sciences, 929*, 105-110.

Penrose, R. (2002). Gravitational collapse: The role of general relativity. *General Relativity and Gravitation, 34*, 1141- 1165.

Penrose, R. (2004). *The road to reality: A complete guide to the laws of the universe*. London: Jonathan Cape.

Penrose, R., and Hameroff, S.R. (1995). What "gaps"? Reply to Grush and Churchland. *Journal of Consciousness Studies, 2*, 98-111.

Perrine, K. R. (1991). Psychopathology in epilepsy. *Seminars in Neurology, 11*, 175-181.

Perry, B. D. (1994). Neurobiological sequelae of childhood trauma: PTSD in children. In M. Murberg, (Ed.), Catecholamines in Post-traumatic Stress Disorder (pp. 233–55). *American Psychiatric Press.*

Pestana, M.S. (2006). Association mechanisms and the intentionality of the mental. *Journal of Mind and Behavior, 27*, 91-120.

Peterson I. (1993). Newton's clock: Chaos in the solar system. W.H. Freeman: New York.

Petitot, J. (2003). The neurogeometry of pinwheels as a sub-Riemannian contact structure. *Journal of Physiology Paris, 97*, 265-309.

Petrovic, P. and Ingvar, M. (2002). Imaging cognitive modulation of pain processing. *Pain, 95*, 1-5.

Petrovic, P., Kalso, E., Petersson, K.M., and Ingvar M. (2002). Placebo and opioid analgesia– imaging a shared neuronal network. *Science, 295*, 1737-40.

Pevet, P., Agez, L., Bothorel, B., Saboureau, M., Gauer, F., Laurent, V., and Masson-Pevet, M. (2006). Melatonin in the multi-oscillatory mammalian circadian world. *Chronobiology International, 23*, 39-51.

Peyron, R., Laurent, B., and Garcia-Larrea, L. (2000). Functional imaging of brain responses to pain. A review and meta-analysis. *Neurophysiologie Clinique, 30*, 263– 288.

Phelps, E.A., O'Connor, K.J., Gatenby, J.C., Gore, J.C., Grillon, C., and Davis, M. (2001). Activation of the left amygdala to a cognitive representation of fear. *Nature Neuroscience, 4*, 437-441.

Phillips, R.G., and LeDoux, J.E. (1992). Differential contribution of amygdala and hippocampus to cued and contextual fear conditioning. *Behavioural Neuroscience, 106*, 274-285.

Ploghaus, A., Narain, C., Beckmann, C.F., Clare, S., Bantick, S., Wise, R., Matthews, P.M., Rawlins, J.N.P., and Tracey, I. (2001). Exacerbation of pain by anxiety is associated with activity in a hippocampal network. *Journal of Neuroscience, 21*, 9896-903.

Ploner, M, Freund, H.J., and Schnitzler, A. (1999). Pain affect without pain sensation in a patient with a postcentral lesion. *Pain, 81*, 211-214.

Poetzl, O. (1960). The Relationship between Experimentally Induced Dream Images and Indirect Vision. *Psychological Issues Monograph, 2*, 46-106.

Porte, H., and Hobson, J. A. (1996). Physical motion in dreams: one measure of three theories. *Journal of Abnormal Psychology, 105*, 329- 335.

Post, R.M., Weis, S. R., and Smith, M. A. (1995). Sensitization and kindling. In M. J. Friedman, D. S. Charney, and A. Y. Deutch (Eds.), *Neurobiological and clinical consequences of stress: From normal adaptation to posttraumatic stress disorder*. Philadelphia: Lipincott-Raven.

Post, R.M. and Weiss, R.B. (1998). Sensitization and kindling phenomena in mood, anxiety, and obsessive-compulsive disorders: The role of serotonergic mechanisms in illness progression. *Biological Psychiatry, 44*, 193-206.

Poulet, J.F. and Hedwig, B. (2007). New insights into corollary discharges mediated by identified neural pathways. *Trends in Neurosciences 30*, 14-21.

Price, D.D. (2000). Psychological and neural mechanisms of the affective dimension of pain. *Science, 288*, 1769-72.

Price, D.D., Barrell, J.J., and Rainville P. (2002). Integrating experiential-phenomenological methods and neuroscience to study neural mechanisms of pain and consciousness. *Consciousness and Cognition, 11*, 593-608.

Prince, M. and Peterson, F. (1908). Experiments in psychogalvanic reactions from co-conscious ideas in a case of multiple personality. *Journal of Abnormal Psychology, 3*, 114-131.

Putnam, F.W. (1984). The Psychophysiologic Investigation of Multiple Personality Disorder. *Psychiatric Clinics of North America, 7*, 31-39.

Putnam, F.W. (1989). *Diagnosis and Treatment Multiple Personality Disorder*. New York, London: The Guilford Press.

Putnam, F.W. (1992). Using hypnosis for therapeutic abreactions. *Psychiatric Medicine, 10*, 51-65.

Putnam, F. (1997). *Dissociation in Children and adolescents. A developmental Perspective*. London, New York: The Guilford Press.

Putnam, F.W. (1995). Investigating multiple personality disorder. *British Journal of Psychiatry, 166*, 122–123.

Putnam, F.W., Guroff, J.J., Silberman, E.K., and Post, B.L. (1986). The clinical phenomenology of multiple personality disorder. Review of 100 recent cases. *Journal of Clinical Psychiatry, 47*, 285-93.

Quattrochi, J. J., Mamelak, A. N., Madison, R. D., Macklis, J. D., and Hobson, J. A. (1989). Mapping neuronal inputs to REM sleep induction sites with carbachol-fluorescent microspheres. *Science, 245*, 984-986.

Quen, J. M. (1986). *Split Minds/Split Brains.* New York: New York University Press.

Rainville, P., Duncan, G.H., Price, D.D., Carrier, B., and Bushnell, M.C. (1997). Pain affect encoded in human anterior cingulate but not somatosensory cortex. *Science, 277*, 968-971.

Rainville, P., Hofbauer, R.K., Paus, T., Duncan, G.H., Bushnell, M.C., and Price, D.D. (1999). Cerebral mechanisms of hypnotic induction and suggestion. *Journal of Cognitive Neurosciences, 11*, 110-125.

Rainville, P., Hofbauer, R.K., Bushnell, M.C., Duncan, G.H., and Price, D.D. (2002). Hypnosis modulates activity in brain structures involved in the regulation of consciousness. *Journal of Cognitive Neuroscience, 14*, 887-901.

Rattiner, L.M., Davis, M., and Ressler, K.J. (2005). Brain-derived neurotrophic factor in amygdala-dependent learning. *Neuroscientist, 11*, 323-33.

Raz, A., Fan, J., and Posner, M.I. (2005). Hypnotic suggestion reduces conflict in the human brain. *Proceedings of the National Academy of Sciences of the United States of America, 94*, 102, 9978-83.

Read, J., Perry, B. D., Moskowitz, A., and Connolly, J. (2001). The contribution of early traumatic events to schizophrenia in some patients: a traumagenic neurodevelopmental model. *Psychiatry, 64*, 319-45.

Reanault, B., Signoret, J.L., Debruille, B., Breton, F. and Bolgert, F. (1989). Brain Potentials Reveal Covert Facial Recognition in Prosopagnosia. *Neuropsychologia, 27*, 905-912.

Redington, D.J. and Reidbord, S.P. (1992). Chaotic dynamics in autonomic nervous system activity of a patient during a psychotherapy session. *Biological Psychiatry, 31*, 993-1007.

Rees, G., Russell, C., Frith, C.D. and Driver, J. (1999). Inattentional blindness versus inattentional amnesia for fixated but ignored words. *Science, 286*, 2504–2507.

Rees, G. (2001). Neuroimaging of visual awareness in patients and normal subjects. *Current Opinion in Neurobiology, 11*, 150-156.

Rees, G., Kreiman, G., and Koch, C. (2002). Neural correlates of consciousness in humans. Nature Reviews. *Neuroscience, 3*, 261-270.

Reeves, A.L. (1997). Autonomic activity in epilepsy: Diagnostic considerations and implications. *Journal of Epilepsy, 10*, 111-6.

Reinders, A.A.T.S., Nijenhuis, E.R.S., Paans, A.M.J., Korf, J., Willemsen, A.T.M., and den Boer, J.A. (2003). One brain, two selves. *Neuroimage, 20*, 2119-2125.

Rickeport, M.M. (1992). The interface between multiple personality, spirit mediumship and hypnosis. *American Journal of Clinical Hypnosis, 34*, 168-77.

Roberts, R.J., Varney, N.R., and Paulsen, J.S. (1990). Dichotic listening and complex partial seizures. *Journal of Clinical and Experimental Neuropsychology, 12*, 448-458.

Roberts, R.J., Gorman, L.L., Lee, G.P., Hines, M.E., Richardson, E.D., Riggle, T.A., and Varney, N.R. (1992). The phenomenology of multiple partial seizure like symptoms without stereotyped spells: An epilepsy spectrum disorder? *Epilepsy Research, 13*, 167-177.

Roberts, R.J. (1993). Commentary; Positive associations among dichotic listening errors, complex partial epileptic-like signs, and paranormal beliefs. *Journal of Nervous and Mental Disease, 131*, 668-671.

Roberts, R.J. (1999). Epilepsy spectrum disorder in the context of mild traumatic brain injury. In N.R. Varney, R.J. Roberts, and N.J. Hillsdale (Eds.), *The Evaluation and Treatment of Mild Traumatic Brain Injury*, Mahwah: Lawrence Erlbaum, 209-247.

Rofe, Y. (2008). Does repression exist? Memory, pathogenic, unconscious and clinical evidence. *Review of General Psychology, 12*, 63-85.

Romei, V., De Gennaro, L., Fratello, F., Curcio, G., Ferrara, M., Pascual-Leone, A., and Bertini, M. (2008). Interhemispheric transfer deficit in alexithymia: a transcranial magnetic stimulation study. *Psychotherapy and Psychosomatics 77*, 175-81.

Rosenbaum, M. (1980). The role of the term schizophrenia in the decline of diagnoses of multiple personality. *Archives of General Psychiatry, 37*, 1383-1385.

Ross, C.A. (1989). Multiple personality disorder: Diagnosis, clinical features, and treatment. New York: J. Wiley and Sons.

Ross, C.A. (2003). *Multiple personality disorder: Diagnosis, clinical features, and treatment.* New York: J. Wiley and Sons.

Rotenberg, V. S. (1992). Sleep and memory II: Investigations on humans. *Neuroscience and Biobehavioral Reviews, 16*, 503-505.

Rubin, N. (2003). Binocular rivalry and perceptual multi-stability. *Trends in Neurosciences, 26*, 289-291.

Ruel, J.M.H.M., and de Kloet, E.R. (1985). Two receptor systems for corticosterone in rat brain: Microdistribution and differential occupation. *Endocrinology, 117*, 2505-2512.

Russr, M.J., Shearin, E.N., Clarkin, J.E., Harrison, K., and Hull, J.W. (1993). Subtypes of self-injurious patients with borderline personality disorder. *American Journal of Psychiatry, 150*, 1869-1877.

Rutter, J., Reick, M., McKnight, S.L. (2002). Metabolism and the control of circadian rhythms. *Annual Review of Biochemistry, 71*, 307-31.

Saenz, D.A., Goldin, A.P., Minces, L., Chianelli, M., Sarmiento, M.I., and Rosenstein, R.E. (2004). Effect of melatonin on the retinal glutamate/glutamine cycle in the golden hamster retina. *FASEB Journal, 18*, 1912–1913.

Sakai, K., Rowe, J.B., and Passingham, R.E. (2002). Active maintenance in prefrontal area 46 creates distractor-resistant memory. *Nature Neuroscience, 5*, 479-84.

Salley, R. D. (1988). Subpersonalities with dreaming functions in a patient with multiple personalities. *Journal of Nervous and Mental Disease, 176*,112-115.

Sannita, W. (2000). Stimulus-specific oscillatory responses of the brain: a time/frequency related coding process. *Clinical Neurophysiology, 11*, 565–583.

Saper, C.B., Lu, J., Chou, T.C., and Gooley, J. (2005). The hypothalamic integrator for circadian rhythms. *Trends in Neurosciences, 28*, 152-7.

Sar, V. and Ross, C. (2006). Dissociative as a confounding factor in psychiatric research. Psychiatric Clinics of North America, 29, 129-44.

Sarrieau, A., Dussaillant, M., and Moguilewsky, M. (1988). Autoradiographic localization of glucocorticosteroid binding sites in rat brain after in vivo injection of [3H]RU 28362. *Neuroscience Letters, 92*, 14–20.

Saunders, P. and Skar, P. (2001). Archetypes, Complexes and Self-Organization. *Journal of Analytical Psychology, 46*, 305-323.

Saver, J.L. and Rabin, J. (1997). The neural substrates of religious experience. *Journal of Neuropsychiatry and Clinical Neurosciences, 9*, 498-510.

Savitz, J., Solms, M., and Ramesar, R. (2006). The molecular genetics of cognition: dopamine, COMT and BDNF. *Genes, Brain and Behavior, 5*, 311-328.

Sawamoto, N., Honda, M., Okada, T., Hanakawa, T., Kanda, M., Fukuyama, H., Konishi, J., and Shibasaki, H. (2000). Expectation of pain enhances responses to nonpainful somatosensory stimulation in the anterior cingulate cortex and parietal operculum/posterior insula: an event-related functional magnetic resonance imaging study. *Journal of Neuroscience, 20*, 7438-45.

Saxe, G. N., Chawla, N., and van der Kolk, B. (2002). Self-destructive behavior in patients with dissociative disorders. *Suicide and Life-Threatening Behavior, 32*, 313-319.

Sayar K, Kose S, Grabe HJ, Topbas M (2005). Alexithymia and dissociative tendencies in an adolescent sample from Eastern Turkey. *Psychiatry and Clinical Neurosciences, 59*, 127-34.

Schachter, D.L., and Tulving, E. (1994). *Memory Systems*. Cambridge, MA: MIT Press 1994.

Scharfetter, C. (1998). Dissociation and schizophrenia. Schizophrenias- a dissociative nosopoietic construct? *Fortschritte der Neurologie-Psychiatrie, 66*, 520-3.

Schell, A.M., Dawson, M.E., Rissling, A., Ventura, J., Subotnik K.L., Gitlin, M.J., Nuechterlein, K.H., 2005. Electrodermal predictors of functional outcome and negative symptoms in schizophrenia. *Psychophysiology, 42*, 483-492.

Schenk, L. and Bear, D. (1981). Multiple personality and related dissociative phenomena in patients with temporal lobe epilepsy. *American Journal of Psychiatry, 138*, 1311-1316.

Schmid, G.B. (1991). Chaos theory and schizophrenia: elementary aspects. *Psychopathology, 24*, 185-98.

Schmitz, E.,B., Robertson, M., M. and Trimble, M. R. (1999). Depression and schizophrenia in epilepsy: social and biological risk factors. *Epilepsy Research, 35*, 59-68.

Schore, A.N. (2001). The effects of early relational trauma on right brain development, affect regulation and infant mental health. *Infant Mental Health Journal 22*, 201-269.

Schore, A.N. (2002). Dysregulation of the right brain: a fundamental mechanism of traumatic attachment and the psychopathogenesis of posttraumatic stress disorder. *Australian and New Zealand Journal of Psychiatry 36*, 9-30.

Schweinberger, S. R. and Burton, A.M. (2003). Covert recognition and the neural system for face processing. *Cortex, 39*, 9-30.

Sel, R. (1997). Dissociation as complex adaptation. *Medical Hypotheses, 48*, 205-208.

Sem-Jacobsen, C. and Torkildsen, A. (1960). Depth recording and electrical stimulation in human brain. In: *Electrical studies on the unanesthetized brain*. Ed. E.R. Ramey and D.S. O'Doherty. New York: Harper and Row.

Servit, Z. and Musil, F. (1981). Prophylactic treatment of posttraumatic epilepsy: results of a long-term follow-up in Czechoslovakia. *Epilepsia, 22*, 315-320.

Shevrin, H. (2001). Event-related markers of unconscious processes. *International Journal of Psychophysiology, 42*, 209-218.

Shibata, S., Cassone, V.M., and Moore, R.Y. (1989) Effects of melatonin on neuronal activity in the rat suprachiasmatic nucleus in vitro. *Neuroscience Letters, 97*, 140–144.

Shin, Y.W., Lee, J.S., Han, O.S., and Rhi, B.Y. (2005). The influence of complexes on implicit learning. *Journal of Analytical Psychology, 50*, 175-90.

Shulman, M.B. (2003). Laterality and psychopathology circa 1976. *Epilepsy and Behavior, 4*, 576-577.

Sierra, M. and Berrios, G.E. (1998). Depersonalization: neurobiological perspectives. *Biological Psychiatry, 44*, 898-908.

Silber, A. (1970). Functional phenomenon: Historical concept, contemporary defense. *Journal of the American Psychoanalytic Association, 180)*, 519-538.

Silberer, H. (1909). Bericht uber eine Methode, gewisse symbolische Halluzinations-erscheinungen hervorzurufen und zu beobachten. *Jahrbuch*, Vol. 1.

Simonneaux, V. and Ribelayga, C. (2003). Generation of the melatonin endocrine message in mammals: a review of the complex regulation of melatonin synthesis by norepinephrine peptides, and other pineal transmitters. *Pharmacological Reviews, 55*, 325–395.

Singer, W. (1989). The role of acetylcholine in use-dependent plasticity of the visual cortex. In M. Steriade, and D. Biesold (Eds.) *Brain Cholinergic Systems*. Oxford: Oxford University Press.

Singer, W. (1993). Synchronization of Cortical Activity and its Putative Role in Information Procesing and Learning. *Annual Review of Physiology 55*, 349-74.

Singer, W. (2001). Consciousness and the Binding Problem. *Annals of the New York Academy of Sciences, 929*, 123-146.

Singer, W. and Gray, C.M. (1995). Visual feature integration and the temporal correlation hypothesis. *Annual Review of Neuroscience, 18*, 555–586.

Silberman, E, Post, R., Nurenberger, J., Theodore, W., and Boulenger, J. (1985). Transient sensory, cognitive, and affective phenomena in affective illness: A comparison with complex partial epilepsy. *British Journal of Psychiatry, 146*, 81-89.

Silverman, D.H., Munakata, J., Emmes, H., Mandelkern, M.A., Hoh, C.K., and Mayer, E.A. (1997). Regional cerebral activity in normal and pathological perception of visceral pain. *Gastroenterology, 112*, 64-72.

Singer, W. and Gray, C.M. (1995). Visual feature integration and the temporal correlation hypothesis. *Annual Review of Neuroscience, 18*, 555–586.

Singer, T., Seymour, B., O'Doherty, J., Kaube, H., Dolan, R.J., and Frith, C.D. (2004). Empathy for pain involves the affective but not sensory components of pain. *Science, 303*, 1157-62.

Skaper, S.D., Ancona, B., Facci, L., Franceschini, D., and Giusti, P. (1998). Melatonin prevents the delayed death of hippocampal neurons induced by enhanced excitatory neurotransmission and the nitridergic pathway. *FASEB Journal, 12*, 725–731.

Skarda, CH.A. and Freeman, W.J. (1987). How Brains Make Chaos in Order To Make Sense of the World. *Behavioural and Brain Sciences, 10*, 161-95.

Smith, P.F. and Darlington, C.L. (1996). The development of psychosis in epilepsy: a reexamination of the kindling hypothesis. *Behavioural Brain Research, 75*, 59–66.

Smith, E.E. and Jonides J. (1999). Storage and executive processes in the frontal lobes. *Science, 283*, 1657-61.

Smith, S.D. and Bulman-Fleming, M.B. (2004). A hemispheric asymmetry for the unconscious perception of emotion. *Brain and Cognition, 55*, 452-7.

Soule, J., Messaoudi, E., and Bramham, C.R. (2006). Brain-derived neurotrophic factor and control of synaptic consolidation in the adult brain. *Biochemical Society Transactions, 34*, 600-4.

Spence, S., Shapiro, D., and Zaidel, E. The role of the right hemisphere in the physiological and cognitive components of emotional processing. *Psychophysiology* 1996, 33, 112-122.

Spenceley, A. and Jerom, B. (1997). Intrusive traumatic childhood memories in depression: A comparison between depressed, recovered and never depressed women. *Behavioural and Cognitive Psychotherapy, 25*, 309-318.

Sperry, R.W. (1968). Hemisphere deconnection and unity in conscious awareness. *American Psychologist, 23*, 723–733.

Spiegel, D., Bierre, P., and Rootenberg, J. (1989). Hypnotic alteration of somatosensory perception. *American Journal of Psychiatry, 146*, 749-54.

Spiegel, D. and Cardena, E. (1991). Disintegrated experience: the dissociative disorders revisited. *Journal of Abnormal Psychology, 100*, 366-376.

Spiegel, D. (1991). Neurophysiological correlates of hypnosis and dissociation. Journal of *Neuropsychiatry and Clinical Neurosciences, 3*, 440-5.

Spiegel, D. (1997). Trauma, dissociation, and memory. *Annals of the New York Acadademy of Sciences 821*, 225-237.

Spiegel, D. (2003). Negative and positive visual hypnotic hallucinations: attending inside and out. *International Journal of Clinical and Experimental Hypnosis, 51*, 130-146.

Spigelman, I., Li, Z., Banerjee, P.K., Mihalek, R.M., Homanics, G.E., and Olsen, R.W. (2002). Behavior and physiology of mice lacking the GABAA-receptor delta subunit. *Epilepsia, 43*, 3–8.

Spitzer, C., Haug, H. J., and Freyberger, H. J. (1997). Dissociative symptoms in schizophrenic patients with positive and negative symptoms. *Psychopathology, 30*, 67-75.

Spitzer, C., Willert, C., Grabe, H., Rizos, T., Moller, B., and Freyberger, H.J. (2004). Dissociation, hemispheric asymmetry, and dysfunction of hemispheric interaction: A transcranial magnetic stimulation approach. *Journal of Neuropsychiatry and Clinical Neurosciences , 16*, 163-169.

Squires, E.J. (1998). Why are quantum theorists interested in consciousness. In S.R. Hameroff, A. Kaszriak, and A.C. Scott (Eds.), *Toward a science of consciousness II: The second Tucson discussions and debates* (pp. 609–618). Cambridge: MIT Press.

Sramka, M., Sedlak, P., and Nadvornik, P. (1977). Observation of kindling phenomenon in treatment of pain by stimulation in thalamus. In: Neurosurgical treatment in psychiatry. Sweet W (ed), Baltimore: University Park Press, p. 651-654.

Stam, C.J. (2005). Nonlinear dynamical analysis of EEG and MEG: Review of an emerging field. *Clinical Neurophysiology, 116*, 2266-2301.

Startup, M. (1999). Schizotypy, dissociative experiences and childhood abuse: relationships among self-report measures. *British Journal of Clinical Psychology, 38*, 333-44.

Stefano, G.B. and Esch, T. (2007). Love and stress. Activitas Nervosa Superior 26:173-4.

Stehle, J., Vanecek, J., and Vollrath, L. (1989). Effects of melatonin on spontaneous electrical activity of neurons in rat suprachiasmatic nuclei: an in vitro iontophoretic study. *Journal of. Neural Transmission, 78*, 173–177.

Stevens, J.R. (1959). Emotional activation of the electroencephalogram in patients with convulsive disorders. *Journal of Nervous and Mental Disease, 128*, 339-351.

Stevens J.R. (1992). Abnormal reinnervation as a basis for schizophrenia: a hypothesis. *Archives of General Psychiatry, 49*, 238-243.

Stevens, J.R. (1999). Epilepsy, schizophrenia and the extended amygdala. *Annals of the New York Academy of Sciences, 156*, 548-561.

Stickgold, R., Rittenhouse, C., and Hobson, J. A. (1994). Dream splicing: A new technique for assessing thematic coherence in subjective reports of mental activity. *Consciousness and Cognition , 3*, 114-128.

Stickgold, R., Hobson, J. A., Fosse, R., and Fosse, M. (2001). Sleep, learning, and dreams: Off-line memory reprocessing. *Science, 294*, 1052-1057.

Stickgold, R., Fosse, R., and Walker, M.P. (2002). Linking brain and behavior in sleep – dependent learning and memory consolidation. *Proceedings of the National Academy of Sciences of the United States of America, 99,* 16519-21.

Stross, L. and Shevrin, H. (1962). Differences in thought organization between hypnosis and the waking state: An experimental approach. *Bulletin of the Meninger Clinic, 26*, 237-247.

Stross, L. and Shevrin, H. (1968). Thought organization in hypnosis and the waking state. *Journal of Nervous and Mental Disease, 147*, 272-288.

Stross, L. and Shevrin, H. (1969). Hypnosis as a method for investigating unconscious thought processes. *Journal of the American Psychoanalytic Association, 17*, 100-135.

Sullivan, R.M. and Gratton, A. (1999a). Lateralized effects of medial prefrontal cortex lesions on neuroendocrine and autonomic stress responses in rats. *Journal of Neuroscience, 19*, 2834-2840.

Sullivan, R.M. and Gratton, A. (1999b). Medial prefrontal cortex, laterality, and stress. *Journal of Neuroscience, 19*, 2834–2840.

Sullivan, R.M. and Gratton, A. (2002). Prefrontal cortical regulation of hypothalamic–pituitary–adrenal function in the rat and implications for psychopathology: side matters. *Psychoneuroendocrinology, 27*: 99–114.

Summerfield, C., Jack, A.I., and Burgess, A.P. (2002). Induced gamma activity is associated with conscious awareness of pattern masked nouns. *International Journal of Psychophysiology, 44*, 93-100.

Tabibnia, G. and Zaidel, E. (2005). Alexithymia, interhemispheric transfer, and right hemispheric specialization: a critical review. *Psychotherapy and Psychosomatics, 74*, 81-92.

Takahashi, O., Motomi, T., and Morimitsu, S. (2003). Influences of an anticholinergic antiparkinsonian drug, parkinsonism, and psychotic symptoms on cardiac autonomic functions in schizophrenia. *Journal of Clinical Psychopharmacology, 23*, 441-447.

Tedeschi, R.G. and Calhoun, L.G. (1996). The Posttraumatic Growth Inventory: measuring the positive legacy of trauma. *Journal of Traumatic Stress, 9*, 455-471.

Tedeschi, R. and Calhoun, L. (2004). Posttraumatic growth: a new perspective on psychotraumatology. *Psychiatric Times, 21(4)*, 58-60.

Teicher, M., Glod, C., Surrey, J., and Swett, C. (1993). Early childhood abuse and limbic system ratings in adult psychiatric outpatients. *Journal of Neuropsychiatry and Clinical Neuroscience, 5*, 301-306.

Teicher, M., Andersen, S.L., Polcari, A., Anderson, C.M., Navalta, C.P., and Kim, D.M. (2003). The neurobiological consequences of early stress and childhood maltreatment. *Neuroscience and biobehavioral reviews, 27*, 3-44.

Teicher, M., Tomoda, A., and Andersen, S.L. (2006). Neurobiological consequences of early stress and childhood maltreatment: Are results from human and animal studies comparable? *Annals of the New York Academy of Sciences, 1071*, 313-323.

Tender, J. and Kramer, M. (1971). Dream recall. *American Journal of Psychiatry, 128*, 3-10.

Thomas, K. and Davies, A. (2005). Neurotrophins: a ticket to ride for BDNF. *Current Biology, 15*, 262-4.

Thompson-Schill, S.L., D'Esposito, M., Aguire, G.K., and Farah, M.J. (1997). Role of the left inferior prefrontal cortex in retrieval of semantic knowledge: a reevaluation. *Proceedings of the National Academy of Sciences of the United States of America, 94*, 14792-7.

Tiengo, M. (2003). Pain perception, brain and consciousness. *Neurological Sciences, 24*, S76-9.

Tirsch, W. S., Stude, Ph., Scherb H., and Keidel M. (2004). Temporal order of nonlinear dynamics in human brain. *Brain Research Reviews, 45*, 79-95.

Toates, F. (2006). A model of the hierarchy of behaviour, cognition, and consciousness. *Consciousness and Cognition, 15*, 75-118.

Tolle, T.R., Kaufmann, T., Seissmaier, T., Lautenbacher, S., Berthele, A., Munz, F., Zieglgansberger, W., Willoch, F., Schwaiger, M., Conrad, B., and Bartenstein P. (1999). Region-specific encoding of sensory and affective components of pain in the human brain: a positron emission tomography correlation analysis. *Annals of Neurology, 45*, 4-7.

Toichi, M., Kubota, Y., Murai, T., Kamio, Y., Sakihama, M., Toriuchi, T., Inakuma, T., Sengoku, A., and Miyoshi, K. (1999). The influence of psychotic states on the autonomic nervous system in schizophrenia. *International Journal of Psychophysiology, 31*, 147-154.

Tonneau, F. (2004). Consciousness outside the head. *Behaviour and Philosophy, 32*, 97-123.

Tononi, G. and Edelman, G.M. (2000). Schizophrenia and the mechanisms of conscious integration. *Brain Research Reviews, 31*, 391-400.

Treede, R.D., Kenshalo, D.R., Gracely, R.H., and Jones, A.K.P. (1999). The cortical representation of pain. *Pain, 79*, 105-111.

Trief, P.M. (1996). Childhood abuse and chronic pain. observations from clinical practice. *Journal of Interpersonal Violence, 11*, 599-608.

Trimble, M.R. (1996). Anticonvulsant-induced psychiatric disorders. The role of forced normalization. *Drug Safety, 15*, 159.

Tsakiris, M., Haggard, P., Franck, N., Mainy, N., and Sirigu A. (2005). A specific role for efferent information in self-recognition. *Cognition, 96*, 215-231.

Ul'yaninskii, L.S. (1995). Emotional stress and extracardiac regulation. *Neuroscience and Behavioral Physiology, 25*, 257-65.

Uysal, N., Ozdemir, D., Dayi, A., Yalaz, G., Baltaci, A.K., and Bediz, C.S. (2005). Effects of maternal deprivation on melatonin production and cognition in adolescent male and female rats. *Neuroendocrinology Letters, 26*, 555-60.

van de Grind, W. (2002). Physical, neural, and mental timing. *Consciousness and Cognition, 11*, 241-64.

van den Top, M., Buijs, R.M., Ruijter, J.M., Delagrange, P., Spanswick, D. and Hermes, M.L. (2001). Melatonin generates an outward potassium current in rat suprachiasmatic nucleus neurones in vitro independent of their circadian rhythm. *Neuroscience, 107*, 99–108.

Van der Hart, O. and Brown, P. (1992). Abreaction Re-evaluated. *Dissociation, 5*, 127-140.

Van der Hart, O. and Friedman, B. (1989). A Reader's Guide to Pierre Janet on Dissociation: A Neglected Intelectual Heritage. *Dissociation, 2*, 3-16.

van der Kolk, B.A. and van der Hart, O. (1989). Pierre Janet and the breakdown of adaptation of adaptation in psychological trauma. *American Journal of Psychiatry, 146*, 1530-40.

van der Kolk, B., Greenberg, M., Boyd, H. and Krystal, H. (1985). Inescapable shock, neurotransmitters and addiction to trauma: Towards a psychobiology of post traumatic stress disorder, *Biological Psychiatry, 20,* 314-325.

Van Erp, T.G., Saleh, P.A., Rosso, I.M., Huttunen, M., Lönnqvist, J., Pirkola, T., Salonen, O., Valanne, L., Poutanen, V.P., Standertskjold-Nordenstam, C.G., and Cannon, T.D. (2002). Contributions of genetic risk and fetal hypoxia to hippocampal volume in patients with schizophrenia or schizoaffective disorder, their unaffected siblings, and healthy unrelated volunteers. *American Journal of Psychiatry*, 159,1514-1520.

Van Putten, M.J.A.M. and Stam, C.J. (2001). Is the EEG really "chaotic" in hypsarrhythmia. *IEEE Engineering in Medicine and Biology Magazine, 20*, 72–79.

Vaitl, D., Lipp, O., Bauer, U., Schüler, G., Stark, R., Zimmerman, M., Kirsch, P. (2002). Latent inhibition in schizophrenia: Pavlovian conditioning of autonomic responses. *Schizophrenia Research, 55*, 147-158.

Varela, F.J., Lachaux, J.P., Rodriguez, E., and Martinerie, J. (2001). The brainweb: Phase synchronization and large-scale integration. *Nature Reviews Neuroscience, 2*, 229–239.

Velazquez, J.L.P., Cortez, M.A., Snead, III O.C., and Wennberg, R. (2003). Dynamical regimes underlying epileptiform events: role of instabilities and bifurcations in brain activity. *Physica D*, 186, 205-220.

Vermetten, E. and Bremner, J.D. (2004). Functional brain imaging and the induction of traumatic recall: a cross-correlational review between neuroimaging and hypnosis. *International Journal of Clinical and Experimental Hypnosis, 52*, 218-312.

Villemure, Ch. and Bushnell, M.C. (2002). Cognitive modulation of pain: how do attention and emotion influence pain processing? *Pain, 95*, 195-199.

Villemure, C., Slotnick, B.M., and Bushnell, M.C. (2003). Effects of odors on pain perception: deciphering the roles of emotion and attention. *Pain, 106*, 101-8.

Vinogradov, S., Kirkland, J., Poole, J.H., Drexler, M., Ober, B.A., Shenaut, G.K. (2002). Both processing speed and semantic memory organization predict verbal fluency in schizophrenia. *Schizophrenia Research, 8*, 171–181.

Vollrath, L. and Welker, H.A. (1988). Day-to-day variation in pineal serotonin N-acetyltransferase activity in stressed and nonstressed male Sprague-Dawley rats. *Life Sciences 42*, 2223–2229.

von der Malsburg, C. and Schneider, W. (1986). A neural cocktail-party processor. *Biological Cybernetics, 54*, 29–40.

von Franz, M. L. (1964). Science and the unconscious. In C.G. Jung (Ed.), *Man and his symbols* (pp. 304-310). New York: Dell Publishing.

von Franz, M. L. (1974). *Number and time: Reflections leading toward a unification of depth psychology and physics.* Evanston: Northwestern University Press.

von Gall, C., Garabette, M.L., Kell, C.A., Frenzel, S., Dehghani, F., Schumm-Draeger, P.M., Weaver, D.R., Korf, H.W., Hastings, M.H., and Stehle, J.H. (2002). Rhythmic gene expression in pituitary depends on heterologous sensitization by the neurohormone melatonin. *Nature Neuroscience, 5*, 234–238.

von Helmholtz, H. (1962). *Helmholtz's treatise on physiological optics* (J. P. C. Southall, Trans.). New York: Dover. (Original work published 1866).

Wager, T.D., Rilling, J.K., Smith, E.E., Sokolik, A., Casey, K.L., Davidson, R.J., Kosslyn, S.M., Rose, R.M., and Cohen, J.D. (2004). Placebo induced changes in fMRI in the anticipation and experience of pain. *Science, 303*, 1162-7.

Wagstaff, G.F., Brunas-Wagstaff, J., Cole, J., Knapton, L., Winterbottom, J., Crean, V., and Wheatcroft, J. (2004). Facilitating memory with hypnosis, focused meditation, and eye closure. *International Journal of Clinical and Experimental Hypnosis, 52*, 435-55.

Walker, E.A., Katon, W.J., Neraze, K., Jemelka, R.P., and Massoth, D. (1992). Dissociation in women with chronic pelvic pain. *American Journal of Psychology, 149*, 534−7.

Walker, M.C., White, H.S., and Sander, J.W. (2002). Disease modification in partial epilepsy. *Brain, 125*, 1937-50.

Walker, E.F. and Diforio, D. (1997). Schizophrenia: a neural diathesis-stress model. *Psychological Review, 104*, 667-85.

Walter, W.G. (1944). Electroencephalography. *Journal of Mental Science, 90*, 64.

Wan, Q., Man, H.Y., Liu, F., Braunton, J., Niznik, H.B., Pang, S.F., Brown, G.M., and Wang, Y.T. (1999). Differential modulation of GABAA receptor function by Mel1a and Mel1b receptors. *Nature Neuroscience, 2*, 401–403.

Wang, L.M., Suthana, N.A., Chaudhury, D., Weaver, D.R., and Colwell, C.S. (2005). Melatonin inhibits hippocampal long-term potentiation. *European Journal of Neuroscience, 22*, 2231–2237.

Warembourg, M. (1975). Radioautographic study of the rat brain and pituitary after injection of 3H dexamethasone. *Cell Tissue Research, 161*, 183–191.

Watkins, H.H. (1993). Ego-state therapy: an overview. *American Journal of Clinical Hypnosis, 35*, 232-40.

Watkins, J.G. and Watkins, H.H. (1979-80). Ego states and hidden observers. *Journal of Altered States of Consciousness, 5*, 3-18.

Watkins, J.G. and Watkins, H.H. (1990). Dissociation and displacement: where goes the "ouch?" *American Journal of Clinical Hypnosis, 33*, 1-21.

Watkins, J.G. and Watkins, H.H. (2000). The psychodynamics and initiation of effective abreactive experiences. *Hypnos, 32*, 60-67.

Wegner, D.M. (1994). Ironic processes of mental control. *Psychological Review, 101*, 34-52.

Weitzenhoffer, A.M. and Hilgard, E.R. (1962). *Stanford hypnotic susceptibility scale*: Form C. Palo Alto: Consulting Psychologists Press.

Wessely, S., Nimnuan, C., and Sharpe, M. (1999). Functional somatic syndromes: one or many? *Lancet, 354*, 936–939.

Wheatley, J., Brewin, C.R., Patel, T., Hackmann, A., Wells, A., Fisher, P., and Myers, S. (2007). "I'll believe it when I can see it": Imagery rescripting of intrusive sensory memories in depression. *Journal of Behavior Therapy and Experimental Psychiatry, 35*, 371-385.

Wheeler, J.A., and Zurek, W.H. (1983). *Quantum theory and measurement*. New Jersey: Princeton University Press.

Wieser, H.G. (1979). The stereoencephalographic correlate of psychical seizures. EEG-EMG *Zeitschrift fur Elektroenzephalographie, Elektromyographie und verwandte Gebiete, 10*, 197-206.

Wilkeson, A., Lambert, M.T., and Petty, F. (2000). Posttraumatic stress disorder, dissociation, and trauma exposure in depressed and nondepressed veterans. *Journal of Nervous and Mental Disease, 188*, 505-9.

Williams, L.M., Bahramali, H., Hemsley, D.R., Hartus, A.W.F., Brown, K., Gordon, E. (2002). Electrodermal responsivity distinguishes ERP activity and symptom profile in schizophrenia. *Schizophrenia Research, 59*, 115-125.

Wittling, W. and Pfluger, M. (1990). Neuroendocrine hemisphere asymmetries: Salivary cortisol secretion during lateralized viewing of emotion-related and neutral films. *Brain and Cognition, 14*, 243-265.

Wolf, P. (1991). Acute behavioural symptomatology at disappearence of epileptiform EEG abnormality. Paradoxical or 'forced' normalization. *Advances in Neurology, 55*, 127-142.

Wolf, P. and Trimble, M.R. (1985). Biological Antagonism and Epileptic Psychosis. *British Journal of Psychiatry, 146*, 272-276.

Wolfe, L.S. and Millet, J.B. (1960). Control of post-operative pain by suggestion under general anesthesia. *American Journal of Clinical Hypnosis, 3*, 109-112.

Wolff, P. H. (1987). *The development of behavioural and emotional states in infancy*. Chicago: University Chicago Press.

Wong, P.S., Shevrin, H. and Williams, W.J. (1994). Conscious and Nonconscious Processes: An ERP Index of an Anticipatory Response in a Conditioning Paradigm Using Visual Masked Stimuli. *Psychophysiology, 31*, 87-101.

Wong, P.S., Bernat, E., Snodgrass, M., and Shevrin, H. (2004). Event-related brain correlates of associative learning without awareness. *International Journal of Psychophysiology, 53*, 217-31.

Woolf, N. and Hameroff, S. (2001). A quantum approach to visual consciousness. *Trends in Cognitive Neuroscience, 5*, 472–478.

World Health Organization (1993). *The ICD-10. Classification of Mental and Behavioural Disorders. Diagnostic Criteria for Research*. Geneva: World Health Organization.

Wortman, C.B., Loftus, E.F., and Marshall, M.E. (1992). Sensation and Perception. In C.B. Wortman, E.F. Loftus and M.E.Marshall (Eds.), *Psychology*. New York: Mc Graw-Hill.

Yalom, I.D. and Lieberman, M.A. (1991). Bereavement and heightened existential awareness. *Psychiatry, 54*, 334-345.

Yates, J.L. and Nasby, W. (1993). Dissociation, Affect, and Network Models of Memory: An Integrative Proposal. *Journal of Traumatic Stress, 6*, 305-326.

Zaccai, G., Massoulié, J., and David, F. (1998). *From cell to brain: The cytoskeleton intra- and inter-cellular communication the central nervous system*. Amsterdam: Elsevier.

Zahn, T., Frith, C., and Steinhauer, S. (1991). Autonomic functioning in schizophrenia: Electrodermal activity, heart rate, pupillography. In S. Steinhauer, J. Gruzelier, and J. Zubin (Eds.), *Handbook of Schizophhrenia*. Elsevier Science.

Zahn, T.P. and Pickar, D. (2005). Autonomic activity in relation to symptom ratings and reaction time in unmedicated patients with schizophrenia. *Schizophrenia Research, 79*, 257-270.

Zahn, T., Jacobsen, L., Gordon, C., McKenna, K., Frazier, J., and Rapoport, J. (1997). Autonomic nervous system markers of psychopatology in childhood-onset schizophrenia. *Archives of General Psychiatry, 54*, 904–12.

Zeise, M.L. and Semm, P. (1985) Melatonin lowers excitability of guinea pig hippocampal neurons in vitro. *Journal of Comparative Physiology, 57*, 23–29.

Zeman, A. (2001). Consciousness. *Brain; 124*(Pt 7):1263-89.

Zlotnik, C., Shea, M.T., Begin, A., Pearlstein, T., Simpson, E., and Costello, E. (1996). The validation of the Trauma Symptom Checklist-40 (TSC-40) in a sample of inpatients. *Child Abuse and Neglect, 20*, 503-510.

INDEX

A

aberrant, 112
abnormalities, 18, 19, 20, 25, 80, 85, 101, 112, 118
abreaction, 11, 98
abuse, 47, 80, 103, 110, 112, 115, 129, 130
ACC, 51, 52, 56, 58
access, 2, 3, 5, 17, 59, 60, 61, 68, 69, 96
accessibility, 41, 47, 114
accidents, 39, 54, 55, 59
accuracy, 79
acetylcholine, 70, 127
action potential, 45
activation, 1, 2, 4, 11, 20, 21, 28, 29, 31, 45, 47, 51, 56, 57, 58, 70, 85, 96, 104, 110, 111, 113, 115, 129
acute, 31, 40, 52, 118
acute stress, 118
adaptation, 31, 40, 101, 106, 123, 126, 131
addiction, 131
adolescents, 121, 123
adrenal gland, 46, 47
adult, 40, 100, 128, 130
adulthood, 40, 100, 109, 114
adults, 14, 24, 96, 101
advertising, 4
affect, 11
affective dimension, 53, 123
affective disorder, 23, 24, 112
age, 66, 110
agents, 23
aid, 81
alexithymia, 30, 104, 114, 125
alien, 120

allodynia, 50, 116
altered state, 20
alternative, 14, 24, 27
alters, 26, 56, 67, 68, 69, 115
ambiguity, 95
ambiguous stimuli, 1, 25
amenorrhea, 31
American Psychiatric Association, 10, 63, 84, 96
American Psychological Association, 101
amnesia, 7, 9, 16, 17, 33, 39, 40, 41, 45, 54, 56, 64, 65, 66, 67, 69, 124
amphetamine, 120
amphibia, 98
amplitude, 71
amygdala, 27, 30, 40, 42, 43, 84, 88, 95, 97, 100, 104, 112, 115, 117, 118, 120, 123, 124, 129
anaesthesia, 14
analgesia, 12, 13, 21, 39, 40, 50, 52, 53, 102, 108, 113, 120, 122
analgesic, 49
analgesics, 52
analytical psychology, 114
anatomy, 22
anger, 40
animal models, 31, 80, 100
animal studies, 130
animals, 15, 31, 40, 45, 50, 65
antagonism, 22
antagonistic, 17
anterior cingulate cortex, 50, 58, 117, 126
anticholinergic, 129
anticonvulsant, 19, 23, 26
anticonvulsants, 95
antidepressants, 23
antithesis, 106

anxiety, 21, 30, 42, 46, 50, 51, 83, 95, 99, 105, 114, 123
anxiety disorder, 46
APA, 84
application, 16, 45, 52, 79
archetype, 76, 90, 118
argument, vii
Aristotelian, 92
arousal, 42, 88, 102
assessment, 56, 58, 83, 121
associations, 17, 34, 51, 81, 85, 87, 125
asylum, 22
asymmetry, 25, 27, 31, 96, 109
atrophy, 47
attachment, 40, 126
attacks, 9
attention, 2, 12, 42, 49, 50, 51, 52, 53, 75, 88, 96, 105, 106, 121, 131
attitudes, 13, 49, 108
attractor, 89
attractors, 82, 89
atypical, 19, 40, 42, 56, 85, 87, 104
auditory cortex, 36
automatisms, 33, 40, 42
autonomic, 21, 28, 29, 31, 85, 88, 99, 104, 110, 111, 124, 129, 130, 131
autonomic activity, 31, 99
autonomic nervous system, 21, 28, 29, 88, 124, 130
autonomous, 35
autonomy, 9, 34
avoidant, 41
awareness, vii, 1, 2, 3, 4, 12, 13, 30, 44, 52, 53, 54, 58, 59, 60, 61, 63, 67, 69, 89, 106, 114, 116, 119, 120, 124, 133, 134

B

Baars, 1, 2, 3, 50, 59, 60, 61, 96
back pain, 109
baroreflex sensitivity, 111
barrier, 55, 75
basal ganglia, 53
BDNF, 42, 46, 47, 97, 100, 120, 126, 130
Beck Depression Inventory (BDI), 85, 97
behavior, viii, 9, 14, 30, 34, 40, 42, 45, 54, 58, 63, 79, 81, 82, 86, 87, 92, 95, 107, 112, 126, 129
beliefs, 125
benefits, 105
bereavement, 59
bifurcation, 71, 81, 87

bifurcation point, 87
bilateral, 27, 31, 58, 84, 88, 102, 117, 121
binding, 3, 36, 44, 73, 74, 75, 77, 99, 118, 126
biological, 10, 22, 35, 41, 44, 66, 77, 92, 96, 108, 109, 126
biological processes, 92
biological systems, 92, 108
bipolar, 14, 23, 109
bipolar disorder, 23, 109
bipolar illness, 14
birth, 64, 66
black, 75
black hole, 75
blackouts, 64, 66
Bleuler, 98
blindness, 21, 97, 124
blocks, 118
blood, 21, 23, 46, 58, 86
blood flow, 58
blood pressure, 21, 86
Bohr, 76
bonding, 110, 111
bone, 59
bone marrow, 59
bone marrow transplant, 59
borderline, 2, 30, 119, 122, 125
borderline personality disorder, 2, 125
bottom-up, 2, 71
brain, vii, viii, 1, 2, 3, 7, 10, 13, 16, 17, 22, 23, 26, 27, 28, 29, 31, 36, 41, 42, 43, 44, 49, 51, 52, 54, 56, 57, 58, 59, 60, 61, 63, 66, 67, 70, 71, 72, 73, 74, 75, 77, 79, 81, 82, 83, 85, 87, 88, 89, 90, 91, 92, 93, 96, 97, 98, 99, 100, 102, 104, 105, 106, 107, 108, 109, 110, 111, 113, 114, 115, 116, 117, 118, 119, 120, 122, 124, 125, 126, 128, 129, 130, 131, 132, 133, 134
brain activity, 56, 58, 85, 97, 131
brain asymmetry, 29, 31
brain chemistry, 57, 109
brain damage, 2, 7, 26
brain development, 126
brain functions, 36, 77, 89, 90, 91, 116
brain stem, 70, 71
brain structure, 31, 36, 42, 52, 97, 124
brainstem, 49, 58
breakdown, 131
Breuer, 11, 21, 101
British, 7, 106, 115, 117, 118, 119, 120, 121, 123, 127, 129, 133
broad spectrum, 19

burn, 121
burst, 70, 71, 72
butterfly, 80

C

calmodulin, 47
cancer, 59
candidates, 28
capacity, 19
cardiac arrhythmia, 21
cardiac autonomic function, 129
cardiovascular, 21, 104
cardiovascular function, 104
case study, 66, 115
catecholamine, 40
catecholamines, 122
cats, 50
causality, 89
causation, 44
cDNA, 119
cell, 17, 47, 134
cell death, 47
central nervous system, 74, 77, 119, 134
cerebellum, 58
cerebral asymmetry, 31
cerebral cortex, 96, 100
cerebral function, 40, 41, 49, 106
cerebral hemisphere, 82, 100
changing environment, 90
channels, 17, 83
chaos, vii, viii, 15, 16, 18, 25, 72, 79, 80, 81, 83, 84,
    85, 86, 87, 88, 89, 91, 93, 97, 99, 105, 106, 114,
    115, 122
chaotic, 3, 18, 25, 64, 70, 71, 72, 75, 77, 79, 80, 81,
    82, 83, 84, 85, 87, 89, 90, 92, 99, 109, 114, 131
chaotic behavior, 64, 82, 84, 87
chemical, 86, 92
child abuse, 19, 40, 80
childhood, 30, 39, 40, 41, 47, 54, 55, 80, 84, 92, 96,
    110, 122, 128, 129, 130, 134
childhood sexual abuse, 55
children, 14, 41, 64, 101, 112, 122
cholinergic, 70, 71
chronic, 18, 23, 28, 40, 47, 52, 55, 56, 57, 66, 96, 97,
    103, 104, 105, 109, 112, 116, 118, 130, 132
chronic pain, 52, 55, 57, 103, 105, 109, 112, 116,
    118, 130
chronic stress, 28, 47
chronobiology, 97

cingulated, 122
circadian, 16, 44, 108, 112, 122, 125, 131
circadian clock, 108
circadian oscillator, 112
circadian rhythm, 44, 125, 131
circadian rhythms, 44, 125
classical, 19, 73, 75, 76, 92
classical mechanics, 75
classification, 20, 39, 63, 105
clinical, 11, 12, 18, 19, 20, 24, 28, 31, 34, 35, 36, 40,
    42, 50, 52, 56, 59, 61, 65, 67, 69, 83, 84, 87, 98,
    102, 103, 105, 107, 110, 113, 115, 117, 121, 122,
    123, 124, 125, 130
clinical depression, 113
clinical trial, 113
clinical trials, 113
closure, 132
clusters, 70
CNS, 31, 43, 46, 47, 53
Co, 98
Coca-Cola, 4
co-conscious, 123
codes, 73
coding, 74, 125
cognition, 16, 45, 46, 47, 49, 57, 71, 74, 79, 85, 87,
    121, 122, 126, 130, 131
cognitive, 3, 4, 10, 11, 12, 13, 16, 17, 19, 20, 25, 29,
    31, 34, 36, 40, 42, 44, 45, 47, 49, 50, 51, 52, 53,
    55, 56, 57, 60, 65, 69, 70, 71, 73, 79, 82, 83, 84,
    85, 86, 87, 90, 92, 100, 101, 105, 108, 111, 114,
    117, 119, 122, 123, 127, 128
cognitive dimension, 13
cognitive function, 10, 16, 36, 73
cognitive level, 70
cognitive map, 45
cognitive process, 25, 31, 60, 88, 100
cognitive processing, 88
cognitive psychology, 119
cognitive science, 114
coherence, 44, 74, 77, 101, 107, 108, 110, 129
cohesiveness, 68
collaboration, 9, 10
collective unconscious, 77
colonoscopy, 105
colorectal, 105
colorectal cancer, 105
combat, 59, 100, 118
communication, 30, 36, 66, 67, 77, 82, 108, 111, 134
community, 57
compatibility, 34

competition, 1, 2, 16, 17, 29, 71, 72, 80, 81, 82, 83, 85, 87, 90, 110
complementarity, 92
complementary, 92
complex partial epilepsy, 127
complex partial seizure, 19, 23, 26, 27, 64, 124
complex regional pain syndrome, 109
complex systems, 87, 100
complexity, 4, 16, 17, 18, 25, 74, 75, 79, 81, 85, 86, 87, 91, 99
complications, 98, 118
components, 13, 22, 30, 40, 49, 53, 57, 65, 68, 69, 70, 112, 127, 128, 130
composition, 17, 86, 106
computation, 109
computers, 122
computing, 105
concentration, 23
conception, 96
conceptual model, 16, 119
conditioning, 97, 123
conductance, 45
configuration, 17
conflict, 4, 20, 41, 50, 51, 56, 57, 66, 76, 77, 82, 83, 85, 105, 124
conformational, 77
conformity, viii, 54, 63
confusion, 56, 80
connectivity, 46, 50, 57, 106
conscious activity, 4
conscious awareness, 11, 13, 34, 42, 58, 65, 69, 128, 129
conscious experiences, 120
consciousness, vii, 1, 2, 3, 5, 9, 10, 12, 13, 14, 16, 19, 20, 22, 30, 33, 34, 37, 39, 41, 43, 44, 47, 49, 50, 51, 52, 53, 55, 57, 58, 59, 60, 61, 63, 66, 67, 68, 69, 73, 74, 75, 76, 77, 88, 89, 90, 91, 92, 93, 96, 97, 99, 102, 103, 106, 110, 111, 113, 115, 120, 122, 123, 124, 128, 130, 133
conservation, 40
consolidation, viii, 42, 45, 46, 100, 128, 129
construction, 1, 90
consumption, 4
contextualization, 68
continuing, 25
continuity, 71
control, 3, 7, 9, 24, 27, 28, 31, 33, 40, 44, 46, 50, 51, 54, 63, 83, 88, 101, 103, 105, 108, 117, 119, 125, 128, 133
control group, 27, 88

controlled, 11, 29, 52, 83, 110, 117
conversion, 10, 20, 21, 117
conversion disorder, 21
Copenhagen, 76
coping strategies, 40
corpus callosum, 30, 82, 99
correlation, 46, 50, 77, 85, 127, 130
correlation analysis, 130
correlations, 75, 115
cortex, 17, 36, 50, 53, 58, 70, 75, 100, 109, 122, 124, 127
cortical, 2, 17, 22, 50, 51, 58, 88, 95, 101, 112, 129, 130
cortical functions, 50
corticosterone, 31, 125
cortisol, 29, 47, 118, 133
creative thinking, 17
creativity, 83, 96, 99
CREB, 42, 46
critical period, 80
critical value, 88
culture, 59
cybernetics, 113, 132
cytoskeleton, 46, 77, 134

D

data analysis, 83, 84, 85
dating, 66
deafness, 108
death, 20, 59, 127
declarative knowledge, 97
declarative memory, 102
defects, 20, 30, 40
defense, 22, 28, 30, 40, 55, 57, 59, 63, 95, 127
defenses, 11
deficit, vii, 30, 36, 104, 125
deficits, vii, 56, 117
definition, 1, 10, 11, 13, 14, 34, 39, 43, 49, 57, 84
degree, 9, 23, 34, 50, 51, 83, 84, 86, 89
degrees of freedom, 81, 86
delirium, 40
delta, 128
delusions, 30, 120
dementia, 33, 34
denial, viii, 25, 54, 63
density, 46
depersonalization, 9, 18, 39, 40, 54, 60, 80
depressed, 46, 50, 101, 128, 133

Index 139

depression, 9, 14, 21, 23, 24, 26, 27, 28, 46, 47, 79, 85, 97, 99, 107, 109, 115, 128, 133
depressive disorder, 26, 48
depressive symptoms, 23, 48
deprivation, 46, 131
determinism, 89
deterministic, 86, 87, 112
developmental disabilities, 113
dexamethasone, 132
diagnostic, 20, 39, 103
Diagnostic and Statistical Manual of Mental Disorders, 63, 96
diathesis-stress model, 132
dielectric, 108
differential diagnosis, 100, 107
differentiation, 46
dimensionality, 17
discharges, 18, 21, 22, 24, 26, 29, 31, 36, 80, 81, 84, 85, 111, 123
discontinuities, 71
discontinuity, 69, 71
discourse, 87
discovery, 105
discrete behavioral states, 70, 80
diseases, 7, 19, 22, 31, 84
disinhibition, 30
disorder, 18, 23, 26, 35, 40, 54, 55, 63, 64, 66, 69, 80, 83, 100, 106, 107, 109, 110, 111, 118, 123, 125, 133
displacement, 133
dissociated state, 11, 72, 80, 90
dissociation, vii, 3, 7, 8, 9, 11, 12, 14, 15, 16, 17, 18, 19, 20, 21, 24, 25, 27, 28, 30, 33, 34, 35, 37, 39, 40, 41, 42, 47, 49, 51, 53, 54, 55, 57, 59, 60, 61, 63, 64, 65, 69, 72, 80, 82, 84, 85, 88, 97, 98, 99, 100, 101, 106, 116, 117, 120, 128, 133
dissociative disorders, 16, 19, 20, 39, 41, 54, 55, 64, 67, 69, 80, 84, 97, 120, 126, 128
dissociative fugue, 3, 56, 60
dissociative identity disorder, viii, 35, 63, 64, 100, 105
dissociative symptoms, 21, 80
distraction, 34, 35, 111
distress, 53, 58, 59
distributed memory, 16
distribution, 1, 50
dominance, 3, 29, 110
dopamine, 27, 98, 110, 120, 126
dopaminergic, 23, 26, 47, 100
dorsolateral prefrontal cortex, 50, 109

dream, 65, 66, 67, 68, 69, 70, 71, 97, 98, 99, 106, 111, 116, 118
dreaming, vii, viii, 5, 55, 63, 65, 67, 68, 69, 70, 71, 72, 107, 110, 114, 125
drug abuse, 96
drug-resistant, 117
drugs, 19, 22, 23, 40
DSM, 20, 35, 39, 63, 96
DSM-III, 39
duality, 92, 121
dynamical system, 86, 95, 107
dynamical systems, 86, 95, 107
dysfunction, 128
dysfunctional, 30
dysregulated, 31
dysregulation, 20, 29, 31, 88, 114
dysregulation, 126

E

ears, 44
eating, 46
eating disorders, 46
ECG, 86
EDA, 27, 84, 86, 87
education, 119
EEG, 17, 18, 19, 20, 21, 23, 24, 26, 36, 73, 83, 85, 86, 92, 95, 99, 101, 102, 103, 105, 106, 107, 112, 116, 117, 118, 119, 128, 131, 133
EEG activity, 18, 23, 24, 26, 84, 107
EEG patterns, 95, 99
efficacy, 23, 52, 56, 110
ego, 12, 17, 34, 44, 55, 61, 64, 67, 69
Einstein, 116
electrical, 26, 27, 45, 50, 86, 108, 117, 126, 129
electrodermal activity, 117
electroencephalogram, 17, 129
electroencephalography, 18
electron, 77
electrophysiological, 19, 25, 27, 106, 112
EMG, 133
emotion, 2, 9, 41, 42, 45, 49, 58, 68, 84, 103, 104, 115, 116, 128, 131, 133
emotional, 4, 5, 9, 10, 16, 20, 27, 28, 29, 31, 34, 39, 40, 41, 43, 46, 49, 53, 55, 56, 57, 60, 68, 70, 102, 112, 116, 118, 122, 128, 133
emotional conflict, 4, 5
emotional distress, 58
emotional experience, 49, 57
emotional processes, 43, 46

emotional responses, 40, 53
emotional state, 16, 133
emotionality, 31
emotions, 9, 10, 11, 30, 34, 41, 60, 97
empathy, 58
encoding, 42, 43, 53, 130
endocrine, 31, 44, 111, 127
endocrine disorders, 111
endocrine glands, 31
endogenous, 2, 44, 46, 50, 96, 98, 108
energy, 10, 11, 25, 40, 75, 108
entanglement, 77
entropy, 74
environment, 16, 36, 49, 51, 63
environmental, 41, 53, 54, 71
environmental conditions, 53
enzymes, 108
epilepsy, 18, 19, 20, 21, 22, 23, 24, 25, 26, 27, 28, 47, 82, 95, 96, 97, 98, 99, 100, 102, 105, 107, 110, 111, 115, 116, 117, 118, 122, 124, 125, 126, 127, 132
epileptic seizures, 21, 22, 24, 97, 101, 105, 113
epileptiform, 21, 72, 80, 112, 131, 133
epileptogenesis, 25, 26
episodic, 41, 45, 122
episodic memory, 122
epistemological, 91
equilibrium, 26, 70
ERP, 5, 99, 133
ERPs, 2
esophageal, 21
etiology, 9, 25, 34, 103
etiopathogenesis, 27, 35
European, 105, 108, 110, 132
event-related potential, 100, 116
event-related potentials, 100
evidence, 1, 2, 11, 13, 14, 15, 19, 21, 23, 25, 26, 27, 29, 30, 36, 40, 41, 42, 45, 46, 49, 50, 55, 57, 59, 60, 61, 67, 68, 69, 70, 71, 72, 73, 74, 80, 83, 84, 88, 92, 96, 102, 107, 108, 109, 112, 115, 117, 125
evolution, 7, 79, 83, 87
exaggeration, 7
examinations, 65
excitability, 26, 31, 45, 70, 105, 134
excitation, 16, 26, 28
exclusion, 58
executive processes, 128
experimental condition, 5, 56
explicit perception, 3
exposure, 31, 41, 97, 133

exposure, 118
extinction, 115
extracellular, 47
eye, 1, 36, 132
eye movement, 36
eyes, 20, 44

F

facial pain, 56, 104
failure, 25, 81, 87
false, 35, 64
familial, 109
fear, 30, 40, 115, 116, 120, 123
fear response, 30
fears, 112
feedback, 107
feelings, viii, 30, 47, 54, 58, 63, 81, 84
females, 39
fetal, 131
fibers, 82
fibromyalgia, 56, 109
films, 133
fire, 70
First World, 11
flow, 36, 50
fluctuations, 71, 86, 89, 92
focusing, 2, 49
forced normalization, 130
forebrain, 49, 70, 71
forgetfulness, 63
fractal structure, 92
fragmentation, 9, 42, 45, 53, 60, 81, 85
free association, 34
freedom, 86
Freeman, 21, 79, 89, 90, 107, 120, 127
freezing, 13, 40
Freud, vii, viii, 10, 11, 21, 33, 101, 110
frontal cortex, 51
frontal lobe, 36, 87, 96, 105, 128
frontal lobes, 36, 128
frustration, 58
fugue, 33, 40, 65, 66
functional architecture, 75
functional imaging, 58
functional magnetic resonance imaging (fMRI), 51, 56, 58, 96, 97, 100, 102, 105, 107, 108, 115, 116, 126, 132

G

GABA, 20, 27, 98
galvanic skin response, 29, 83
gastrointestinal, 21, 39, 53
gene, 45, 46, 119, 132
gene expression, 45, 46, 119, 132
general anesthesia, 133
general relativity, 122
generalization, 26
generation, 19, 45, 65, 90
genes, 110
genetic, 47, 131
genetics, 126
gland, 44, 46
glucocorticoid receptor, 46, 119
glucocorticoids, 47
glutamate, 46, 125
glutamine, 125
goal-directed, 90
goals, 51, 90
grandparents, 66
gravitation, 122
gravitational field, 75
gravity, 76, 77, 91
grey matter, 50
groups, 18, 73, 74, 75
growth, 46, 59, 101, 130
growth factor, 46
guidance, 90
gyrus, 36, 88

H

hallucinations, 9, 36, 39, 40, 54, 60, 65, 128
hamartomas, 102
handedness, 110
hands, 44
Harvard, 97, 109, 112, 119
head, 26, 130
head trauma, 26
headache, 55
health, 30, 105
hearing, 102
heart, 22, 59, 85, 134
heart attack, 59
heart disease, 22
heart rate, 85, 134
heat, 50, 56, 116

hedonic, 59
Heisenberg, 92, 110
hemisphere, 3, 27, 29, 82, 133
hemispheric asymmetry, 128
heuristic, 75, 77, 93
high-frequency, 96
Hilgard, 111, 133
hippocampal, 19, 40, 43, 45, 100, 102, 104, 111,
     115, 123, 127, 131, 132, 134
hippocampus, 26, 40, 42, 43, 45, 46, 47, 84, 88, 97,
     106, 109, 120, 121, 123
Hippocampus, 104, 119, 120
HIV, 59
holistic, 83
homeostasis, 103
homogeneous, 71
hopelessness, 41, 57, 60
hormones, 29, 105
hospital, 9, 66
hospitalization, 41, 52
hospitalizations, 66
host, 64, 65, 67
HPA axis, 40
human, vii, 1, 7, 12, 18, 26, 41, 54, 58, 59, 63, 72,
     76, 77, 78, 80, 83, 87, 90, 91, 93, 97, 98, 102,
     109, 110, 111, 112, 113, 116, 117, 119, 122, 124,
     126, 130
human brain, viii, 54, 58, 63, 87, 98, 102, 116, 117,
     119, 124, 126, 130
human cognition, 80
human development, 7
human experience, 77
human subjects, 18
humans, 15, 26, 45, 50, 96, 97, 124, 125
hyperalgesia, 97
hyperarousal, 28
hypersensitivity, 80
hypertension, 22
hypnosis, vii, viii, 3, 5, 9, 11, 12, 13, 16, 33, 43, 50,
     51, 52, 53, 54, 55, 59, 60, 65, 66, 68, 69, 70, 102,
     103, 106, 110, 114, 120, 123, 124, 128, 129, 131,
     132
hypnotic, 5, 12, 14, 43, 50, 51, 52, 55, 56, 59, 64, 65,
     67, 84, 92, 98, 99, 100, 102, 113, 124, 128, 133
hypochondria, 24
hypothalamic, 26, 31, 102, 114, 125, 129
hypothalamus, 97
hypothesis, 2, 17, 24, 25, 26, 27, 28, 34, 44, 55, 57,
     59, 60, 61, 68, 69, 77, 80, 83, 88, 91, 96, 100,
     103, 111, 127, 129

hypoxia, 98, 131
hysteria, 7, 9, 10, 21, 24, 33, 34, 41, 65, 98, 101
hysterical neurosis, 64

I

IASP, 112
ICD, 20, 40, 41, 64, 134
ice, 13
idealization, 77, 91
identity, vii, 2, 10, 17, 20, 29, 35, 39, 41, 52, 53, 54,
    60, 63, 64, 69, 80, 100, 107
illusion, 115
imagery, 2, 108
images, 1, 5, 53, 60, 68, 70, 71, 89, 90, 121
imagination, 44, 106
imaging, 2, 19, 27, 102, 106, 122, 131
immobilization, 46
implicit knowledge, 12
implicit memory, 12
implicit perception, 3
in situ, 58
in vitro, 111, 127, 129, 131, 134
in vivo, 109, 118, 126
inactivation, 23, 28
incest, 103
incidence, 23, 26, 27, 98
induction, 42, 45, 56, 118, 124, 131
infancy, 133
information processing, viii, 4, 13, 17, 50, 51, 54,
    63, 68, 69, 75, 87, 117
inhibition, 9, 21, 26, 28, 30, 39, 53, 85, 131
inhibitory, 20, 25, 26, 27, 28, 33, 40, 45, 47, 51, 57,
    70
initiation, 79, 87, 133
injection, 83, 126, 132
injury, 41, 54, 56, 120
insertion, 30
insight, 10
insomnia, 46, 113
instabilities, 75, 131
instability, 80, 83, 86, 87, 96
insults, 41, 113
integration, 2, 11, 30, 31, 36, 40, 43, 44, 53, 55, 57,
    59, 60, 61, 65, 67, 69, 70, 73, 74, 83, 88, 89, 90,
    96, 120, 127, 130, 131
integrity, 36, 37, 42, 59, 61, 64
intelligence, 17
intensity, 2, 50, 52, 69, 71, 83, 102
intentional archetypes, 89

intentionality, 122
intentions, 30
interaction, 28, 46, 50, 76, 82, 92, 128
interaction, 29
interactions, 2, 21, 36, 44, 68, 69, 74, 89, 92
interdisciplinary, vii, 86
interface, 115, 122, 124
interference, 71, 83, 85, 88, 116
international, 57
interpretation, 3, 28, 52, 54, 57, 59, 60, 61, 76
intervention, 117
interview, 20, 103, 109
intoxication, 40
intracranial, 27, 95, 116
intrinsic, 45, 120
introspection, 3
intrusions, 19
intuition, 90
invasive, 50
investigations, 125
ipsilateral, 27
irritability, 20, 85, 99

J

Jackson, 118
JAMA, 110
Janet, 10, 21, 110, 112, 131
Jung, vii, viii, 9, 12, 15, 33, 34, 65, 68, 77, 90, 91,
    98, 110, 113, 132
Jungian, 117

K

Kant, 106
kinase, 46
kinases, 47
kindling, 80, 123, 127
kinesthetic, 21, 39, 53

L

language, 76, 77, 91
large-scale, 44, 131
latency, 5
laterality, 28, 29, 83, 111, 129
law, 77
laws, 79, 90, 93, 122

lead, vii, 1, 4, 5, 9, 11, 18, 20, 21, 25, 28, 30, 33, 40, 41, 42, 44, 47, 53, 54, 55, 57, 60, 65, 68, 71, 75, 77, 79, 80, 81, 82, 83, 85, 87, 90, 91, 92
learned helplessness, 41
learning, 15, 16, 45, 59, 70, 89, 90, 111, 116, 122, 124, 127, 129, 133
learning process, 70
left hemisphere, 19, 27, 28, 29, 88
lesions, 56, 119, 129
libido, 10
limbic system, 20, 21, 22, 25, 26, 29, 51, 89, 130
linear, 89, 95, 116
links, 72, 77, 85, 87
listening, 124, 125
literature, 23, 30, 34, 67, 69, 72
lobectomy, 13, 98
localization, 46, 126
location, 109
locus, 40, 70
locus coeruleus, 40, 70
long-term, 40, 42, 45, 46, 95, 102, 113, 115, 118, 119, 121, 126, 132
long-term impact, 40
long-term memory, 42
long-term potentiation, 42, 45, 46, 95, 102, 115, 118, 121, 132
love, 40, 106
low back pain, 56, 104
LTP, 45, 46, 104
Lyapunov exponent, 83, 84, 85, 88

M

macrosystem, 86
magnetic resonance imaging (MRI), 100, 109
magnetic resonance spectroscopy, 109
maintenance, 51, 68, 125
major depression, 121
maladaptive, 31
malignant, 11
maltreatment, 130
mammals, 127
management, 59, 105
mania, 14
manic, 23, 26
manipulation, 2, 56, 111
MAPK, 47
mapping, 102
Markov, 71
materialism, 91

maternal, 45, 66, 131
mathematical, 75, 76, 77, 79, 81, 90, 91, 93
mathematical knowledge, 91
mathematics, 76, 77, 78, 81, 91
matrix, 58
meanings, 96
measurement, 3, 4, 76, 83, 84, 85, 88, 100, 133
measures, 28, 58, 83, 85, 87, 92, 97, 129
mechanical, 76, 86
mechanics, 76, 114, 117
medial prefrontal cortex, 31, 42, 103, 129
medication, 22, 23
medications, 23, 40
medicine, 55, 116
meditation, 132
MEG, 102, 128
melancholic, 101
melatonin, 44, 45, 46, 97, 98, 101, 107, 108, 111, 115, 118, 121, 125, 127, 129, 131, 132
memory, vii, 7, 9, 11, 13, 15, 16, 20, 30, 36, 39, 40, 41, 42, 43, 44, 45, 46, 47, 51, 53, 54, 55, 60, 65, 66, 69, 70, 73, 83, 84, 97, 99, 101, 102, 103, 104, 115, 116, 119, 120, 125, 128, 129, 132
memory deficits, 97
memory formation, 45, 46, 47, 119
memory loss, 53
memory processes, vii, 42
mental activity, 9, 129
mental disorder, 46, 79, 87
mental health, 126
mental illness, 24
mental image, 2, 80, 90
mental imagery, 2
mental processes, 10, 79, 87, 88, 92
mental representation, 12, 16, 17, 18, 28, 36, 73, 80, 81, 82, 85
mental representations, 80
mental state, 14, 17, 21, 22, 52, 53, 81, 82, 92, 119
mental states, 14, 17, 81, 82, 119
mesoscopic, 90
messages, 4
meta-analysis, 120, 122
metabolic, 28, 45
metabolite, 46
metaphor, 44, 97
metaphors, 57
mice, 115, 128
microcosm, 76
microscopy, 46
microspheres, 124

microstructure, 16
microtubule, 77
microtubules, 109, 110
midbrain, 50, 110
migraine, 96
migraines, 110
migraineurs, 96
mind, 72, 89
mind-body, 10, 112
mind-body problem, 10
mineralocorticoid, 119
minority, 52
mirror, 26, 90
misidentified, 37
misinterpretation, 60
MIT, 110, 117, 118, 119, 126, 128
mitogen, 47
modality, 44
modeling, 17
models, 16, 50, 51, 69, 81, 108, 115, 116
modulation, 13, 27, 42, 45, 49, 50, 52, 53, 54, 55, 56, 59, 84, 88, 110, 111, 122, 131, 132
molecular mechanisms, 47
molecules, 47
momentum, 86
mood, 15, 16, 26, 46, 58, 81, 92, 109, 122, 123
motion, 2, 98, 108, 123
motivation, 58
motor activity, 36
motor area, 36
motor control, 21, 39, 53, 122
motor function, 73
motor system, 106
motor task, 16
mouse, 111, 121
movement, 36, 71, 75
MPD, 69, 80
mPFC, 31
multidimensional, 14, 49, 86
multiple personality, viii, 3, 7, 9, 12, 13, 14, 17, 18, 20, 28, 33, 34, 35, 39, 40, 41, 54, 55, 60, 61, 63, 64, 65, 66, 67, 68, 69, 80, 83, 95, 97, 98, 100, 101, 103, 107, 110, 111, 116, 118, 119, 121, 123, 124, 125
multiple personality disorder, viii, 7, 9, 12, 14, 17, 18, 20, 28, 33, 34, 35, 39, 41, 54, 55, 61, 63, 64, 65, 67, 68, 69, 80, 83, 97, 100, 107, 110, 116, 118, 119, 121, 123, 124
multiplicity, 91
mystical experiences, 14

N

N-acety, 109, 132
narratives, 114
National Academy of Sciences, 97, 102, 104, 108, 112, 113, 119, 120, 124, 129, 130
natural, 39, 50, 79
natural laws, 79
nausea, 52
negative emotions, 42
negative mood, 98
negative valence, 41
neglect, 40
Nemiah, 120
neocortex, 23, 26, 47
nerve, 51, 120
nerve growth factor, 120
nervous system, 44, 46, 114, 134
network, 16, 17, 18, 21, 42, 45, 53, 56, 57, 58, 100, 121, 122, 123
neural assemblies, 80
neural function, 56
neural mechanisms, 85, 123
neural network, 16, 17, 25, 52, 69, 70, 71
Neural Network Model, 116
neural networks, 16, 17
neural systems, 16, 87
neuroanatomy, 96
neurobiological, 16, 18, 24, 25, 27, 40, 42, 69, 92, 93, 112, 127, 130
neurobiology, 102, 106
neurodegeneration, 97
neurodegenerative, 47
neurodegenerative disorders, 47
neurodynamics, 107
neuroendocrine, 28, 29, 31, 44, 108, 129
neuroendocrine system, 108
neurohormone, 132
neuroimaging, 42, 54, 102, 131
neurologist, 7
neuromodulation, 114
neuronal excitability, 15
neuronal plasticity, 106
neurons, 16, 17, 18, 20, 26, 44, 46, 47, 70, 71, 73, 74, 75, 77, 88, 89, 96, 103, 113, 127, 129, 134
neurophysiological circularity, 90
neuroscience, vii, viii, 73, 74, 79, 90, 91, 93, 97, 111, 116, 123
neurotic, 34
neurotransmission, 127

neurotransmitter, 47
neurotransmitters, 131
neurotrophic, 42, 46, 98, 120, 124, 128
neutral stimulus, 4
new, vii, viii, 7, 10, 12, 15, 17, 33, 42, 43, 46, 59,
    68, 69, 70, 71, 73, 75, 79, 81, 84, 85, 86, 87, 89,
    93, 95, 100, 102, 103, 108, 110, 119, 122, 129,
    130
Niels Bohr, 92
nightmares, 68, 69
NMDA, 45
nociception, 49, 57, 102
nociceptive, 13, 49, 51, 53, 56, 57, 103
noise, 71
non-human, 50
non-human primates, 50
nonlinear, 3, 15, 75, 79, 81, 83, 85, 88, 89, 90, 91,
    92, 100, 106, 130
non-linear, 71
non-linear, 75
non-linear, 90
non-linear, 122
nonlinear dynamic systems, 15
nonlinear dynamics, 86, 106, 130
norepinephrine, 27, 127
normal, 1, 7, 10, 13, 14, 19, 20, 22, 26, 30, 31, 34,
    41, 45, 47, 53, 55, 60, 65, 70, 84, 85, 87, 104,
    123, 124, 127
normalization, 22, 23, 24, 27, 99, 115, 121, 130, 133
nuclei, 70
nucleus, 70, 74

O

observations, 28, 40, 76, 83, 92, 95, 130
obsessive-compulsive, 123
obsessive-compulsive disorder, 123
occupational, 88
odors, 131
opioid, 122
optics, 132
orbitofrontal cortex, 51
ordering factors, 90
organ, 89
organic, 25, 26, 40, 41, 66
organism, 3, 22, 50, 86, 92
organization, viii, 5, 18, 55, 65, 66, 68, 71, 80, 82,
    85, 87, 90, 92, 104, 122, 129, 132
oscillation, 71, 114
oscillations, 17, 74, 81, 106, 115

oscillatory activity, 88
outpatients, 130
overload, 87

P

P300, 5
pain, vii, viii, 12, 13, 14, 21, 39, 40, 41, 47, 49, 50,
    51, 52, 53, 54, 55, 56, 57, 58, 59, 60, 95, 96, 102,
    103, 104, 105, 106, 107, 109, 110, 111, 112, 117,
    118, 119, 121, 122, 123, 126, 127, 128, 130, 131,
    132, 133
pain management, 52
pain reduction, 53
panic attack, 83, 99, 109, 112, 118
panic disorder, 83, 101, 109
paper, 73, 101
paradox, 76
parallel distributed processing model, 18
paranoid schizophrenia, 28
parasympathetic, 28, 40, 96
parasympathetic nervous system, 40
parental influence, 19
parietal lobe, 88
parkinsonism, 129
partial seizure, 19, 27, 31, 104, 124
passive, 28, 40
pathogenesis, 24, 47, 87
pathogenic, 125
pathology, 24, 26, 30, 56, 80
pathophysiological, 24, 87
pathophysiology, 83, 87
pathways, 2, 14, 31, 36, 47, 51, 60, 123
patients, 1, 3, 5, 13, 18, 19, 20, 21, 22, 23, 24, 26,
    27, 28, 30, 34, 35, 37, 39, 46, 47, 52, 53, 54, 55,
    57, 60, 63, 64, 68, 69, 80, 82, 83, 84, 85, 88, 99,
    101, 104, 109, 112, 118, 124, 125, 126, 129, 131,
    134
Pavlovian, 131
Pavlovian conditioning, 131
PDP, 16, 17, 18, 81, 118
pelvic, 55, 96, 132
pelvic pain, 55, 96, 132
peptides, 127
perception, vii, 1, 2, 3, 4, 9, 21, 25, 36, 39, 49, 53,
    54, 57, 73, 96, 98, 102, 105, 106, 107, 116, 118,
    127, 128, 130, 131
perceptions, 52, 57, 60, 74, 98
performance, 46, 51, 112
perfusion, 42

personal, 14, 49, 54, 56, 59, 63
personal identity, 54, 56
personality, vii, 7, 11, 12, 13, 14, 17, 28, 29, 34, 35, 39, 42, 44, 54, 55, 63, 64, 65, 66, 67, 68, 69, 80, 83, 90, 95, 98, 100, 101, 103, 109, 111, 115, 118, 123, 125, 126
personality disorder, 17, 28, 39, 54, 55, 63, 64, 66, 69, 70, 80, 100, 103, 109, 118, 125
PET, 36, 102
PET scan, 36
PFC, 42, 43, 51, 84
pharmacodynamics, 105
pharmacological, 49, 95
phase transitions, 86
phenomenology, 96, 101, 124
philosophical, 76, 77, 91, 92, 115
philosophy, 59, 110
phobia, 4
physical abuse, 39, 110
physical world, 77, 78, 91, 93
physics, 73, 86, 91, 92, 122, 132
physiological, 9, 26, 28, 29, 34, 40, 42, 44, 52, 53, 64, 65, 69, 86, 103, 106, 110, 111, 121, 128, 132
physiology, 43, 72, 86, 96, 107, 128
pig, 134
pilot study, 100
pineal, 44, 46, 97, 108, 127, 132
pineal gland, 44, 46, 97
pinealocyte, 46, 119
pituitary, 31, 110, 111, 115, 129, 132
pituitary gland, 31
placebo, 50
plasma, 31
plasticity, 15, 45, 46, 95, 127
Plato, 76
play, 9, 18, 24, 41, 44, 47, 51, 64, 68, 69, 78, 84
plurality, 35
Poincaré, 79, 86
poison, 76
polycystic ovarian syndrome, 31
polypeptide, 46
Pontogeniculoocipital system, 70
poor, 88
population, 19, 23, 40, 41, 117
positive correlation, 51
positron emission tomography, 104, 130
post traumatic stress disorder (PTSD), 9, 41, 47, 84, 100, 107, 118, 121, 122, 123, 126, 131,
postsynaptic, 20
Posttraumatic Growth Inventory, 130

post-traumatic stress, 17, 39, 100, 118, 123, 126
potassium, 45, 131
predictability, 79, 117
prediction, 79
predictors, 126
predisposing factors, 22
pre-existing, 89, 90
pre-existing chaotic fluctuations, 89
prefrontal cortex, 31, 45, 50, 57, 58, 108, 118, 129, 130
pregnancy, 68
preservative, 40
pressure, viii, 54, 63, 86
presynaptic, 75
primary visual cortex, 2, 75, 103
probability, 17, 75
problem solving, 88
processing stages, 105
production, 30, 33, 46, 67, 119, 131
production function, 67
prognosis, 104
prolactin, 115
property, 16
prophylactic, 26
proposition, 83
prosopagnosia, 99
protein, 42, 46
protein synthesis, 42, 46
proteins, 77
prototype, 65, 69, 80, 97
psyche, 9, 33, 34, 63, 65, 90, 91, 113
psychiatric disorders, 27, 40, 121, 130
psychiatric illness, 115
psychiatric patients, 27, 57, 112
psychiatry, 22, 33, 57, 59, 108, 115, 121, 128
psychic process, 65, 91
psychoanalysis, 10, 11, 118
psychobiology, 131
psychogenic, 20, 21, 33, 39, 41, 54, 65, 66
psychological, vii, 7, 8, 9, 13, 16, 30, 33, 35, 40, 41, 42, 49, 53, 57, 65, 72, 77, 80, 81, 85, 89, 90, 91, 93, 112, 131
psychological pain, 57
psychological phenomena, 9
psychological processes, vii, 13
psychological stress, 40, 41
psychological stressors, 40
psychologist, 7
psychology, 10, 57, 59, 68, 79, 91, 93, 97, 107, 117, 132

psychopathology, 7, 10, 22, 26, 27, 46, 84, 101, 127, 129

psychophysiological, 72, 85, 92

psychoses, 19, 96

psychosis, 21, 22, 24, 26, 27, 109, 115, 120, 121, 127

psychosomatic, 20, 22, 92, 109, 111, 116, 118

psychosurgery, 103

psychotherapeutic, 43

psychotherapy, 10, 42, 59, 100, 124

psychotic, 22, 23, 24, 27, 28, 34, 64, 129, 130

psychotic states, 28, 130

psychotic symptoms, 22, 24, 64, 129

Putnam, 11, 29, 69, 80, 98, 123

Q

quantization, 76

quantum, 73, 75, 76, 77, 91, 92, 93, 97, 106, 110, 117, 128, 133

quantum dynamics, 97

quantum entanglement, 77

quantum fluctuations, 92

quantum gravity, 76, 77

quantum mechanics, 73, 76, 93, 106, 117

quantum phenomena, 92

quantum state, 77

quantum theory, 76, 77, 93

questionnaire, 120

R

R and D, 39

rain, 90

random, 3, 22, 79, 85, 87, 112

randomness, 79, 85, 86

range, 21, 108

raphe, 70, 103

rapid eye movement sleep(REM sleep), 69, 70, 71, 102, 105, 124, 102

rat, 46, 105, 108, 113, 120, 125, 126, 127, 129, 131, 132

ratings, 50, 52, 130, 134

rats, 46, 50, 95, 97, 115, 117, 129, 131

reaction time, 34, 134

realism, 77, 93

reality, 12, 75, 76, 91, 122

recall, 14, 15, 42, 43, 47, 63, 84, 92, 99, 130, 131

recalling, 10

receptors, 20, 46, 108, 120, 132

reciprocity, 23, 26

recognition, 105, 126

reconditioning, 42

reconsolidation, 42, 43, 84, 104

recovery, 88, 112

recurrence, 66

reduction, 9, 52, 53, 76, 77, 81, 91, 92, 108, 110, 116

reference frame, vii, 54, 63

reflection, 59, 67, 69, 70, 72, 108

refractory, 23, 118

regional, 50

regression, 117

regular, 85

regulation, 31, 45, 46, 52, 102, 124, 126, 127, 129, 131

rejection, 105

relationship, vii, 15, 17, 18, 19, 20, 21, 22, 23, 25, 26, 27, 28, 30, 31, 33, 45, 47, 48, 50, 52, 55, 56, 57, 67, 68, 69, 72, 83, 85, 100, 106, 111

relationships, 55, 59, 65, 129

relativity, 75, 76, 77, 93, 122

relaxation, 84, 96

relaxation time, 96

relevance, 15, 27, 108

reliability, 98

religion, 59

religious, 20, 90, 126

repression, 9, 10, 11, 25, 68, 82, 101, 125

reprocessing, 42, 44, 84, 129

research, vii, 3, 7, 11, 12, 13, 16, 22, 31, 34, 36, 42, 43, 49, 51, 57, 59, 68, 69, 74, 77, 84, 85, 86, 90, 92, 113, 118, 121, 125

research reviews, 113

researchers, 102

resistance, 4, 66

resolution, 59, 68

respiratory, 21

responsiveness, 14, 19, 25, 50

restoration, 12, 68

retardation, 113

retina, 98, 125

retrograde amnesia, 7, 41

rheumatoid arthritis, 59

rhythmicity, 44

rhythms, 44, 81, 107

right hemisphere, 28, 29, 83, 95, 110, 111, 128

risk, 96, 109, 114, 126, 131

risk factors, 114, 126

rodents, 50

S

sample, 126, 134
scalp, 19, 21
schemas, 47
schizoaffective disorder, 23, 131
schizophrenia, 22, 26, 27, 28, 30, 33, 34, 35, 36, 46,
    47, 64, 79, 85, 87, 96, 98, 99, 100, 103, 104, 105,
    106, 107, 108, 109, 110, 116, 117, 120, 121, 122,
    124, 125, 126, 129, 130, 131, 132, 133, 134
schizophrenic, 109, 116, 128
schizophrenic patients, 22, 23, 35, 64, 88, 109, 111,
    116, 117, 128
schizotypy, 119
school, 11
science, 91, 93, 110, 122, 128
scientific, 7, 10, 73, 76, 90, 91, 103
scientific knowledge, 103
scientific theory, 91
SCN, 45, 114, 118
scores, 58
search, 103, 106
Second World War, 12, 35
secretion, 29, 46, 101, 133
sedation, 52
segregation, 14
seizure, 18, 19, 20, 21, 23, 24, 26, 29, 66, 67, 71, 83,
    95, 109, 113, 124
seizures, 18, 20, 21, 22, 23, 24, 25, 26, 28, 39, 66,
    80, 95, 102, 104, 105, 106, 107, 113, 133
selecting, 51
selective attention, 1, 117
self, 9, 36, 52, 60, 65, 66, 70, 74, 90, 114, 126
self-awareness, vii, 54, 63
self-help, 12, 13, 55, 61
self-identity, 37
self-monitoring, 36, 67, 70, 108
self-organization, vii, viii, 3, 70, 71, 75, 77, 79, 80,
    81, 86, 87, 92, 97
self-organizing, 71, 89, 90, 92, 114
self-recognition, 60, 131
self-reflection, 59
self-report, 129
semantic, 85, 87, 121, 130, 132
semantic memory, 85, 87, 132
semantic processing, 87
sensation, 13, 21, 39, 44, 53, 56, 123
sensations, 44, 47, 56
sensing, 54

sensitivity, vii, 15, 19, 27, 52, 79, 80, 84, 92, 108,
    109
sensitization, 10, 19, 26, 27, 47, 132
sensorimotor cortex, 58
sensory experience, 56
sensory systems, 36, 51, 89, 106
separation, 14, 45
sequelae, 122
series, 14, 121
serotonergic, 47, 70, 123
serotonin, 27, 120, 132
sexual abuse, 14, 39, 54, 59, 103, 112
sexually abused, 67, 69, 96
shame, viii, 41, 54, 63, 118
shape, 68, 69
shares, 5, 68
shock, 131
short period, 79
short-term, 42, 88
short-term memory, 42
siblings, 131
side effects, 113
signaling, 45, 46, 51
signaling pathways, 45, 46
signals, 2, 36, 44, 50, 52, 54, 57, 58, 60, 73, 74, 115
signs, 26, 125
simulation, 88
sites, 124, 126
skills, 11
skin, 4, 50, 109
skin conductance, 109
sleep, 16, 46, 67, 69, 70, 71, 105, 111, 124, 129
sleep disturbance, 46
social, vii, 40, 50, 54, 57, 63, 88, 102, 105, 116, 121,
    126
social care, 40
social environment, vii, 50, 57, 116
social exclusion, 58, 105
social relations, 57
social relationships, 57
sodium, 28
solar system, 122
solutions, 80
somatic symptoms, 20, 40
somatization, 96
somatoform, 21, 53, 120
somatosensory, 50, 53, 56, 58, 100, 124, 126, 128
sounds, 102
spacetime, 122
space-time, 76, 89, 90

spatial, 46, 47, 73, 110
spatial memory, 46
spatiotemporal, 45, 90
specialists, 21
specialization, 16, 108, 129
specificity, 56
spectrum, vii, 21, 54, 63, 95, 104, 111, 125
speculation, 106
speech, 36, 87, 107, 116, 117
speed, 75, 132
speed of light, 75
spheres, 34
spinal cord, 71
spine, 108
spiritual, 59
spirituality, 59
Sprague-Dawley rats, 132
stability, 3, 52, 71, 99, 119, 125
stabilize, 44
statistical analysis, 88
status epilepticus, 97
stimuli, 133
stimulus, 1, 2, 3, 4, 5, 14, 26, 50, 51, 56, 58, 89, 100
stochastic, 88, 97, 107, 114
storage, 30, 46, 108
strategies, 40, 55, 60, 80
stream of consciousness, 12
streams, 9, 12
strength, 8, 12, 18, 45, 81
stress, viii, 16, 18, 19, 20, 21, 25, 27, 28, 29, 31, 35,
    39, 41, 42, 45, 46, 47, 54, 56, 57, 59, 64, 84, 85,
    95, 96, 97, 99, 100, 101, 103, 108, 110, 111, 119,
    122, 123, 129, 130, 131, 132, 133
stressful events, 19, 25, 83
stressors, 19, 25, 40
stress-related, 19, 26, 31, 45
structural equation model, 101
structure, 69, 113
students, 119
subcortical structures, 24, 42, 51
subjective, 2, 44, 52, 53, 58, 74, 76, 83, 92, 102, 119,
    129
subjective experience, 2, 44, 52, 74, 83, 102, 119
subjectivity, 119
subliminal perception, 4, 68, 114
substance abuse, 96
substrates, 119, 126
suffering, 13, 18, 52, 58, 68, 69
suicidal, 121
superimposition, 1

superposition, 16, 76
suppression, 17, 28, 50, 96
suprachiasmatic nuclei, 44, 129
suprachiasmatic nucleus, 108, 110, 112, 113, 127,
    131
surgery, 13
surgical, 23, 28, 30, 102
survival, 46
survivors, 110
susceptibility, 113, 133
switching, vii, 54, 56, 63, 70, 88
symbols, 65, 68, 90, 132
sympathetic, 28, 84, 88
symptom, 133, 134
symptoms, 9, 11, 18, 19, 20, 21, 22, 23, 24, 25, 26,
    27, 30, 34, 35, 36, 39, 40, 41, 53, 55, 56, 57, 59,
    61, 64, 80, 83, 85, 87, 97, 105, 112, 120, 124,
    126, 128
synapses, 46
synaptic plasticity, 45, 46, 47, 100
synaptic strength, 17, 45
synaptic transmission, 45, 121
synchronization, 36, 44, 73, 74, 77, 88, 95, 131
synchronous, 74, 81, 88
syndrome, 19, 66, 106, 118
synthesis, vii, 47, 73, 77, 106, 111, 127
systems, 9, 26, 27, 28, 30, 40, 42, 43, 45, 47, 70, 81,
    86, 88, 89, 92, 93, 95, 106, 111, 116, 125

T

target stimuli, 100
task performance, 101
teens, 66
temperature, 86
temporal, 18, 19, 20, 22, 23, 25, 26, 27, 28, 31, 36,
    41, 44, 45, 67, 83, 85, 98, 106, 107, 111, 116,
    117, 118, 119, 126, 127
temporal lobe, 18, 19, 20, 22, 23, 25, 26, 27, 31, 36,
    67, 84, 98, 106, 107, 111, 117, 118, 119, 126
temporal lobe epilepsy, 19, 20, 22, 23, 26, 107, 111,
    117, 126
temporolimbic epilepsy, 28, 95
tension, 9, 70
thalamus, 26, 50, 53, 56, 128
theoretical, vii, viii, 64, 75, 87, 93, 107, 115
theory, vii, viii, 7, 10, 11, 12, 14, 15, 28, 34, 47, 57,
    65, 67, 70, 71, 74, 75, 76, 77, 83, 86, 87, 90, 91,
    93, 100, 105, 112, 120, 122, 126, 133
therapeutic, 10, 11, 23, 43, 55, 83, 84, 123

therapeutic practice, 55
therapeutic process, 11
therapy, 22, 23, 24, 26, 43, 52, 64, 65, 67, 69, 72, 84,
    97, 132
thermal, 104
thermodynamics, 86
thinking, 17, 36, 63, 106
threat, 40, 112
threatened, 40, 55, 59
threatening, 41, 58
three-dimensional, 17
threshold, 5, 13, 16, 54, 55, 59, 71, 95, 105
thresholds, 81
time series, 85, 114, 116
timing, 131
tissue, 26, 49, 52, 56, 57
tolerance, 121
top-down, 2
tradition, 12, 59
training, 103
transcendent function, 90, 113
transcranial magnetic stimulation, 125, 128
transcription, 42, 46
transcription factor, 42, 46
transcription factors, 42
transfer, 30, 104, 125, 129
transference, 60
transformation, 43, 68, 84
transition, 14, 76
transitions, 15, 71, 79, 83, 88, 92
transmission, 45, 46, 47, 49, 82
transportation, 59
trauma, 9, 14, 18, 19, 26, 30, 40, 41, 54, 55, 59, 65,
    67, 68, 69, 80, 84, 85, 101, 105, 106, 110, 114,
    120, 122, 126, 130, 131, 133
traumatic brain injury, 125
traumatic event, 11, 47, 124
traumatic events, 9, 14, 34, 39, 40, 54, 84, 124
traumatic experiences, vii, 33, 65
travel, 56
trend, 53
trial, 100, 115
TSC, 134
tunneling, 75
tunneling effect, 75
turbulence, 115
tyrosine, 46

U

unconscious, 90
unconscious perception, 128
undergraduate, 119
undifferentiated schizophrenia, 66
unification, 132
unilateral, 27, 96, 116
universe, 122
urinary, 21, 118

V

validation, 115, 134
values, 14, 86
variability, 85, 106
variable, 89
variables, 14
variation, 109, 132
vegetables, 65
velocity, 75
verbal abuse, 40
verbal fluency, 132
veterans, 100, 133
victims, 19, 41, 54, 80, 103
violence, 109
virtual reality, 121
visible, 79
vision, 108
visual, 1, 2, 3, 36, 70, 73, 75, 96, 98, 101, 102, 104,
    115, 121, 124, 127, 128, 133
visual attention, 2, 104
visual field, 3
visual processing, 98
visual system, 102
voice, 66
vomiting, 52
vulnerability, 19

W

waking, 14, 66, 67, 69, 70, 71, 114, 129
water, 13
web, 89
Werner Heisenberg, 92
William James, 9
withdrawal, 30, 40
witness, 13
women, 31, 96, 110, 111, 128, 132

working memory, 51, 96, 113
World Health Organization, 64, 134
World War, 11
writing, 12, 13